中国医疗体制改革中基本药物政策的效果评价

Effect Analysis of National Essential Medicine System in China

卞鹰　　　　主编
宋燕　殷实　副主编

山东大学出版社

图书在版编目(CIP)数据

中国医疗体制改革中基本药物政策的效果评价:英
文/卞鹰主编.—济南:山东大学出版社,2020.8
ISBN 978-7-5607-6695-9

Ⅰ.①中⋯　Ⅱ.①卞⋯　Ⅲ.①药品管理－方针政策－
研究－中国－英文　Ⅳ.①R954

中国版本图书馆 CIP 数据核字(2020)第 167102 号

策划编辑　唐　棣
责任编辑　张申华
封面设计　王　艳

出版发行　山东大学出版社
社　　址　山东省济南市山大南路 20 号
邮政编码　250100
发行热线　(0531)88363008
经　　销　新华书店
印　　刷　济南巨丰印刷有限公司
规　　格　720 毫米×1000 毫米　1/16
　　　　　17.25 印张　376 千字
版　　次　2020 年 8 月第 1 版
印　　次　2020 年 8 月第 1 次印刷
定　　价　70.00 元

Preface

Although China embraced the concept of essential medicines in 1979, it still lacked a comprehensive national essential medicine policy during the first decade of the 21st century. In the most recent health care reform (2009-2011), Chinese government proposed the establishment of National Essential Medicine System (NEMS). It was designed to make essential medicine available, control drug prices and reduce irrational drug use. This book makes a comprehensive analysis on the effect of NEMS in China. It consists of two parts.

Part I is aimed to assess its effects on policy objectives and provide reflections for the way forward. It firstly summarizes the recent attempts of China's NEMS and constructs a framework for assessment, and evaluates its implementation in China. Empirical data were obtained through questionnaire survey and prescriptions and documents review conducted in rural primary health centers (PHCs) from four provinces (Shandong, Zhejiang, Anhui and Ningxia) during 2010-2011. Key informant interview and focus group discussion were also used.

Results shows a median decrease of 34.38% in price was witnessed between 2009 and 2010. The declines were also recorded in the mean number of drugs prescribed per patient (from 3.64 to 3.46) and the proportion of patients being prescribed antibiotics (from 60.26% to 58.48%). Increases in the utilization of essential medicines have occurred. The availability of essential medicines reached 66.83% at PHCs. The facilities' income structure has been changed and the proportion of drug income decreased. A high satisfaction towards NEMS was expressed by stakeholders. However current medicine prices remain high compared to international reference prices. Medicines are often unaffordable for poor residents. The new shortage of some drugs occurs. Over-prescription of antibiotics and injections as well as poly-pharmacy remain common compared to WHO standards. Importantly, most PHCs encounter substantial financial losses. The compensation of health care providers for NEMS-related reductions was largely ineffective.

To conclude, NEMS is mostly headed in the right direction and impact on access to and rational use of medicines. The remaining poor outcomes might be indicative of problems in policy design and implementation. China now needs to address gaps and challenges to reach its stated reform goals. Policy implications are discussed.

Part II is to investigate the outpatient medicine use in the rural area of China, monitoring the status of rational use of medicines (RUM), and identifing the organizational barriers of health institutions on the achievement of RUM by establishing a comprehensive evaluation method for RUM outcomes. It also attempts to provide some policy recommendations and suggestive strategies based on the results.

Four provinces (Zhejiang, Anhui, Shandong and Ningxia) with different socio-economic status were selected as study regions to carry out field study on the effect of the NEMS on RUM from 2009 to 2011. To conduct analysis on RUM at the in-depth stage of healthcare reform, the outpatient prescriptions were sampled with randomization from three tiers of health institutions: village health care clinics (VHCs), township heath centers (THCs), county-level hospitals (CHs), in the rural area of 7 provinces (Gansu, Guangxi, Guizhou, Ningxia, Sichuan, Xizang and Xinjiang) of western China in 2012.

Descriptive statistics were used to represent the RUM status by SDUIs, and the results were compared with the WHO reference standard. Pre-post comparative study around implementation of the NEMS was conducted with ANOVA and chi-square test. PCA was used to establish a comprehensive method for evaluating the overall RUM status. Univariate analysis and multivariate regression were used to identify the organizational barriers associated with the achievement of RUM.

After the NEMS implementation, the amount of total medicines and antibiotics used per prescription dropped and the number of essential medicines used per prescription increased in the four provinces. The percentage of prescriptions with injections declined in all the four provinces, but the percentages of prescriptions with antibiotics or hormones were different in different areas. Compared with the WHO reference standard, the RUM status after the NEMS implementation was not up to the policy goal.

Almost every derived indicator in outpatient prescriptions from the health institutions in every sample region or at every organizational level was worse than that of the WHO standard. Excess use of medicines remained prevalent, and improper polypharmacy and use of antibiotics and injections were the main impediment to RUM achievement.

The organizational barriers associated with the RUM achievement differed among different tiers of health institutions in rural areas. Firstly, the RUM status in town-run VHCs was evidently better than that in the VHCs with any other ownership. Secondly, overstaffed health workers led to irrational use of medicines in the VHCs and the THCs. Thirdly, the more health workers received relevant training, the better the RUM status was in the THCs. Last but not least, adopting separation of revenue and expenditure budgets could not lead to reaching the policy goal; instead, it did adverse impact on the RUM achievement in the THCs and the CHs.

To conclude, the RUM status was unsatisfactory after the implementation of the NEMS and at in-depth stage of thenew healthcare reform. Actions should be taken to promote the strategies that help RUM to remove the organizational barriers.

Contents

Part I

Chapter 1 Introduction ··· (6)

   1.1 General background ································· (6)

   1.2 Specific background ······························· (20)

   1.3 Research goals and objectives ····················· (27)

   1.4 Research methodology and design ··················· (28)

   1.5 Potential contributions ···························· (30)

   1.6 Design and organization ··························· (31)

Chapter 2 Theoretical and methodological consideration ··············· (33)

   2.1 Definition of items ······························· (33)

   2.2 Program logic model of China's NEMS ··············· (34)

   2.3 Theory and method of policy evaluation ············· (37)

   2.4 Indicators for monitoring essential medicines policy ······ (40)

   2.5 Fieldwork design ································· (49)

   2.6 Other methods used in this research ················ (51)

Chapter 3 Current progress on the implementation of China's NEMS ··· (53)

   3.1 Overall progress in implementation ················ (53)

   3.2 Essential medicine list ···························· (54)

   3.3 Centralized procurement ·························· (56)

   3.4 Distribution and delivery ·························· (58)

3.5　Compensation for zero-profit policy ·················· (58)

3.6　Summary ·· (59)

Chapter 4　Impact on medicine prices and affordability ·········· (61)

4.1　Materials and methods ·································· (61)

4.2　Results ·· (64)

4.3　Discussion ·· (74)

4.4　Summary ·· (76)

Chapter 5　Effect on improving rational drug use ············· (77)

5.1　Materials and methods ·································· (77)

5.2　Results ·· (79)

5.3　Discussion ·· (84)

5.4　Summary ·· (87)

Chapter 6　Impact on primary health-care facilities ············· (88)

6.1　Introduction ·· (88)

6.2　New characteristic of primary health-care facilities under NEMS
··· (89)

6.3　Tentative compensation for primary care facilities: a SD approach
··· (93)

6.4　Discussion ·· (113)

6.5　Summary ·· (116)

Chapter 7　Awareness, perception and satisfaction among stakeholders ······ (117)

7.1　Materials and method ·································· (117)

7.2　Results ·· (119)

7.3　Discussion ·· (123)

7.4　Summary ·· (125)

Chapter 8　Conclusion and policy recommendation ·········· (126)

8.1　Conclusion ·· (126)

8.2　Policy recommendation ································ (128)

References ·· (133)

Appendices ·· (144)

   Appendix I: Questionnaire of hospital general information ········ (144)

   Appendix II: Questionnaire of medicine prices ····················· (145)

   Appendix III: Questionnaire of satisfaction on NEMS for rural residents
   ··· (146)

   Appendix IV: Questionnaire of satisfaction on NEMS for primary
          health workers ·· (149)

   Appendix V: Interview outline ····································· (151)

Part II

List of Abbreviations ··· (155)

Chapter 1　Introduction ·· (157)

   1.1　Background ·· (157)

   1.2　Research objectives ··· (164)

   1.3　Potential contributions ··· (164)

   1.4　Design and organization ·· (165)

Chapter 2　Literature Review ··· (168)

   2.1　The concept of RUM ·· (168)

   2.2　The specifications of RUM ··· (171)

   2.3　Summary of irrational use of medicines ························ (173)

   2.4　Interventions to promote RUM ·································· (179)

   2.5　NEMS and RUM ··· (184)

   2.6　The SDUIs ·· (194)

Chapter 3　Methodology ·· (203)

   3.1　Research objectives ··· (203)

   3.2　Research design ·· (204)

   3.3　Data source ·· (205)

   3.4　Sampling and data collection ······································ (208)

3.5 Data processing and analysis ·· (209)

Chapter 4 Result I: The Effect of the NEMS on RUM ·················· (215)

4.1 Total medicines prescribed per encounter ······················· (215)

4.2 EMs use ·· (216)

4.3 Antibiotics use ·· (216)

4.4 Injections use ··· (218)

4.5 Hormones use ··· (219)

4.6 Discussion ··· (220)

Chapter 5 Result II: Establishment of a Comprehensive Evaluation
Method for RUM ·· (223)

5.1 The status of medicine use at the in-depth stage of the NHCR
··· (223)

5.2 Establishment of a comprehensive evaluation model ·········· (229)

5.3 Discussion ··· (235)

Chapter 6 Result III: Organizational Barriers Associated with the
Achievement of RUM ··· (239)

6.1 Organizational barriers associated with the achievement of RUM
in VHCs ·· (239)

6.2 Organizational barriers associated with the achievement of RUM
in THCs ·· (241)

6.3 Organizational barriers associated with the achievement of RUM
in CHs ··· (244)

6.4 Discussion ··· (246)

Chapter 7 Conclusion ·· (250)

7.1 Policy recommendation ·· (250)

7.2 Limitations ·· (252)

7.3 Perspectives of future work ··· (253)

References ·· (254)

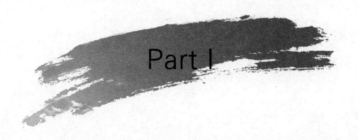

Part I

List of Abbreviations

ADR	Adverse Drug Reaction
ALOS	Average Length of Stay
ANAPE	Average Number of Antibiotics Prescribed per Encounter
ANDPE	Average Number of Drugs Prescribed per Encounter
AR	Arrival Rate of Medicines
ATM	Access to Medicines
CPA	Centralized Procurement Agency, India
CPI	Consumer Price Index
DMC	Drug Management Cycle
DSPRUD	Delhi Society for the Promotion of Rational Use of Drugs, India
DSM	Dynamic Synthesis Methodology
EMs	Essential Medicines
EML	Essential Medicine List
EMLC	Essential Medicine List for Children
GDP	Gross Domestic Product
GMP	Good Manufacturing Practices
HAI	WHO Health Action Initiative on Essential Medicines
HO	Hospital Operation
ICER	Incremental Cost-effectiveness Ratio
INRUD	International Network for the Rational Use of Drugs
IRMSF	Increase Rate of Medical Service Fee

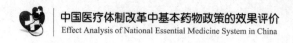
IRP	International Reference Price
KAP	Knowledge-Attitude-Practice
LIP	Low-income Population
MIP	Middle-income Population
MoH	Ministry of Health
MOHRSS	Ministry of Human Resources and Social Security
MPR	Median Price Ratio
MSD	Medical stores department, Tanzania
MSH	Management Sciences for Health
NED	National Essential Drug
NEMS	National Essential Medicine System
NEML	National Essential Medicine List
NRCMS	New Rural Cooperative Medical Services
NRDC	National Reform and Development Commission
OECD	Organization for Economic Cooperation and Development
PBAC	Pharmaceutical Benefits Advisory Committee
PBPA	Pharmaceutical Benefits Pricing Authority
PBS	Pharmaceutical Benefits Schedule
PEA	Percentage of Encounters with an Antibiotic Prescribed
PED	Provincial Supplement Essential Drug
PEH	Percentage of Encounters with Hormone Prescribed
PEI	Percentage of Encounters with an Injection Prescribed
PEM	Percentage of Drugs Prescribed from National Essential Medicine List
PEML	Provincial Supplemented Essential Medicines List
PHC	Rural Primary Health Center
PHW	Primary Health Worker
PPP	Purchasing Power Parity
PSF	Pharmaceutical Service Fee
RDU	Rational Drug Use

RR	Response Rate of Medicine Delivery
SD	System Dynamics
SES	Socio-economic Status
SFDA	State Food and Drug Administration
SR	Subsidy Rate
STGs	Standard Treatment Guidelines
TCM	Traditional Chinese medicine
TFDA	Tanzania Food and Drug Authority
TMC	Total Medical Cost per Patient Visit
UNHCR	United Nations High Commissioner for Refugees
UNICEF	United Nations Children's Fund
WHA	World Health Assembly
WHO	World Health Organization
WMs	Western Medicines

Chapter 1　Introduction

1. 1　General background

1. 1. 1　Essential medicines: the great health reform

The essential medicine concept, a major breakthrough in health care, started in 1977 when World Health Organization (WHO) published its first list and since then it quickly became part of the global public health vocabulary. Essential medicine has been regarded as the most cost-effective element of public health after immunization and key health promotion habits (Quick et al., 2002), and yet, access to essential medicines is now considered a universal human right (WHO, 2013b).

1. 1. 1. 1　Concept of essential medicines

According to the definition of WHO, essential medicines (EMs) are those that satisfy the priority health care needs of the population. (WHO, 2002a) They are selected with due regard to public health relevance, evidence on efficacy and safety, and comparative cost-effectiveness. Essential medicines are intended to be available within the context of functioning health systems at all times in adequate amounts, in the appropriate dosage forms, with assured quality and adequate information, and at a price the individual and the community can afford. (WHO, 2013a)

In 1978, the Declaration of Alma Ata identified "provision of essential drugs" as one of the eight elements of primary health care. (WHO, 2003a) The 1985 Nairobi conference resulted in the development of essential medicines strategy, in which the emphasis was moved beyond selection of drugs to their procurement, distribution, rational use, and quality assurance; and also stressed their validity for industrialized countries. (WHO, 1987)

However, the implementation of the concept of essential medicines is flexible and adaptable to many different situations. There is a misunderstanding that essential medicines are "cheap", instead of the best choice of medicine . Experience has shown that careful selection of a limited range of essential medicines results in a higher quality of care, better management of medicines, and a more cost-effective use of available health resources. (Kar, Pradhan & Mohanta, 2010)

1.1.1.2 Rationale behind the establishment of essential medicine concept

The manufacture of medicines on an industrial scale is about 100 years old. The appearance of antibiotics in the late 1930s led to a revolution in health care and made it possible to treat diseases which until then had been considered fatal. (WHO, 2013c) Since then, tens of thousands of pharmaceutical specialties were flooding the markets as the result of the proliferation of commercial variations of the same active ingredients. In spite of this surfeit, most of the population was unable to afford the medicines needed to address the most basic needs, as their prices and marketing were decided with an affluent population in mind. (Mamdani, 1992) The background to this was marked by failure to select medicines, unfettered advertising, a chaotic drug distribution system, a lack of objective information on medicines and weak or non-existent regulatory agencies. (Halfdan, 2009) In the 1960s and 1970s, in response to skyrocketing expenditure on medicines, various developing countries initiated policies to rationalize medicine expenditure in order to ensure wider and better access. Countries such as Peru, Sri Lanka, Egypt, Cuba and Costa Rica identified the development of national lists of priority medicines, bulk procurement and local manufacture as the channels for responding to the imbalance that existed. (Mamdani, 1992)

The World Health Assembly of 1975 was a watershed. This Assembly introduced the concepts of "essential drugs" and "national drug policy", and hoped to close the huge gap between those who were benefiting from the pharmaceutical harvest of the mid-1900s and those who could not access these medicines. (WHO, 2003a) It began developing this bridge based on pioneering efforts by countries as diverse as Papua New Guinea, Peru, Sri Lanka, and Tanzania. It meanwhile requested WHO to develop means to assist Member States in formulating and implementing national drug policies. This resolution was followed by the First WHO Model List of Essential Medicines in 1997 as well as a series of events that marked the evolution of country essential medicine programmes with the assistance of WHO.

1.1.2 Essential medicines policy

The essential medicines policy is directly linked to the concept of essential medicines and also called national essential medicine system (NEMS). For both of them, the principal point of reference is the primary health care model. The adoption of NEMS is a government commitment to promote the efficient management of pharmaceuticals and support country to close the access gap. It provides a framework within which the activities of the pharmaceutical sector can be coordinated.

1.1.2.1 Origins at national level

Countries implement the essential medicine systems always for three main reasons. The first reason is access including affordability. Medicines can be one of the largest expenses among poor families and contribute to poverty. In these settings, essential medicine programmes have been used to ensure access. In some developed countries, the introduction of new medicines is one of the most important drivers of increasing healthcare costs. Careful selection of the most cost-effective essential medicines is undertaken for procurement and reimbursement in order to achieve the best possible health outcomes for the lowest possible costs. The second reason is rational use. In worldwide there exists at the same time problems of underuse of cost-effective medicines as well as over-prescription of unnecessary medicines. These problems can be prevented through the promotion of essential medicines. The third reason is quality and safety. Consumers and patients are unable to judge the quality and safety of the production of medical products. They have to rely on the strength of the systems for regulatory approval and quality assurance for medicines. (Helen , 2013)

Therefore, although strategies for NEMS may differ from country to country depending on the specific political, economic and social situations and the health status, the overall policy objectives of NEMS recognized throughout the world include to ensure: (1) access: equitable availability and affordability of essential drugs; (2) quality: the quality, safety and efficacy of all medicines; (3) rational use: the promotion of therapeutically sound and cost-effective use of drugs by health professionals and consumers. (WHO, 2003c)

    1.1.2.2   Key strategies of NEMS

    Regarding the system design, the key components of NEMS recommended by WHO include selection of EMs, affordability, financing, supply, quality assurance, rational use, research, human resources and monitoring. (WHO, 1995) Table 1-1 indicates how they relate to the three main objectives of NEMS and that most components cannot be linked to one objective only. (WHO, 2003c)

Table 1-1   Components of a national essential medicine system, linked to key policy objectives (WHO, 2003c)

Components	Objectives		
	Access	Rational use	Quality
Selection of EMs	X	X	(X)
Affordability	X		
Drug financing	X		
Supply systems	X	(X)	
Regulation and quality assurance		X	X
Rational use		X	
Research	X	X	X
Human resources	X	X	X
Monitoring and evaluation	X	X	X

X=direct link; (X) =indirect link

(1)*Selection of EMs*. Drug selection, preferably linked to national clinical guidelines, is a crucial step in ensuring access to essential drugs and in promoting rational drug use, because no public sector or health insurance system can afford to supply or reimburse all drugs that are available on the market. Key policy issues are: the adoption of essential medicine concept to identify priorities for government involvement in the pharmaceutical sector, especially for drug supply in public sector and for reimbursement schemes; procedures to define and update the national list of essential drugs; and selection mechanisms for traditional and herbal medicines.

(2) *Affordability*. Affordable prices are an important prerequisite for ensuring access to essential drugs. Key policy issues are: for all drugs, pricing policy and reduction of drug taxes, tariffs and distribution margins; for multi-source products, promotion of competition through generic substitution and good procurement practices; for single-source products, price negotiations, competition through price information and therapeutic substitution, and TRIPS-compliant measures.

(3) *Drug financing*. It is another essential component to improve access to essential drugs. Key policy issues are: measures to improve efficiency and reduce waste; increased government funding for priority diseases, and the poor and disadvantaged; promotion of drug reimbursement as part of public and private health insurance schemes; use and scope of user charges as a drug financing option; use of and limits of development loans for drug financing; guidelines for drug donations.

(4) *Supply systems*. The fourth essential component of strategies to increase access is a reliable supply system. Key policy issues are: public-private mix in drug supply and distribution systems; commitment to good pharmaceutical procurement practices in public sector; publication of price information on raw materials and finished products; drug supply systems in acute emergencies; inventory control; and disposal of unwanted or expired drugs.

(5) *Regulation and quality assurance*. Key policy issues are: government commitment to drug regulation; independence and transparency of the drug regulatory agency; definition of current and medium-term registration procedures; commitment to good manufacturing practices (GMP), inspection and law enforcement; commitment to regulation of drug promotion; regulation of traditional and herbal medicines; need and potential for systems of adverse drug reaction monitoring; international exchange of information.

(6) *Rational use*. Efforts to promote rational drug use should also cover the use of traditional and herbal medicines. Key policy issues are: development of evidence-based clinical guidelines, as the basis for training, prescribing,

drug utilization review, drug supply and drug reimbursement; establishment and support of drugs and therapeutics committees; promotion of the concepts of essential drugs, rational drug use and generic prescribing in basic and in-service training of health professionals; consumer education, and ways to deliver it; financial incentives to promote rational drug use; regulatory and managerial strategies to promote rational drug use.

(7) *Research*. There are two categories of research that are of particular importance in the development and implementation of NEMS. Operational research is aimed at better understanding of factors affection drug use, and identifying the best methods of selecting, procuring, distributing and using drugs. Drug research and development includes a broad range of activities, including research into new drugs, drugs for neglected infectious diseases, new dosage forms and manufacturing processes; basic research in chemistry and molecular biology; and clinical and field trials of drugs and vaccines.

(8) *Human resources*. It includes the policies and strategies chosen to ensure that there are enough trained and motivated personnel available to implement the components of NEMS. Key policy issues are: government responsibility for planning and overseeing the development and training of human resources needed for pharmaceutical sector; definition of minimum education and training requirements for each category of staff; career planning and team building in government service; the need for external assistance (national and international).

(9) *Monitoring and evaluation*. Key policy issues are: explicit government commitment to the principles of monitoring and evaluation; monitoring of the pharmaceutical sector through regular indicator-based surveys; independent external evaluation of the impact of NEMS on all sectors of the community and the economy.

1.1.3 WHO Model List of Essential Medicines

Since 1977, the WHO has produced a Model List of Essential Medicines which is revised every two years. Its contents are not mandatory and it is, however, as its name suggests, an indicative list. Consequently, the medicines included in it are not equally "essential" to all countries; the list rather provides a basis to enable countries to adopt their own national lists. The structure of the Model List has remained largely unchanged since first published; medicines are divided into two categories: core, defined as efficacious, safe, and cost-effective medicines for priority conditions (selected on the basis of current and estimated future public-health relevance and potential for safe and cost-effective treatment); and complementary, defined as "medicines for priority diseases which are efficacious and safe but not necessarily affordable or less attractive cost-effectiveness in a variety of settings, or for which specialized health care facilities or services may be needed" (WHO, 2002a, 2011c).

The Model List is prepared by the WHO Expert Committee on the Use of Essential Drugs, and then approved by the Director-General of WHO. The Committee is comprised of eight to twelve members drawn from WHO Advisory Panels for Drug Evaluation and for Drug Policies and Management, nine taking into account regional representation (Halfdan, 2009). In drawing up the list, an effort is made to maintain a balance between the Committee's necessary independence and the broad participation of interested parties (industry, patients' groups and the authorities). From 1999 onwards, the selection process for medicines in the Model List evolved from expert evaluation to an evidence-based approach. (WHO, 2001)

The first WHO Model List contained 216 molecules including duplicates and 204 molecules excluding duplicate listings.[1] In May 2007, the World Health Assembly adopted resolution WHA 60.20 Better Medicines for Children, setting goals and calling for action by Member States and WHO to address the global need for children's medicines. (WHO, 2007a) The first Essential Medicines List for Children (EMLC) was then issued by WHO in October 2007. It is intended for use for children up to 12 years of age and is the most significant addition to the Model List. The current versions are the 18th WHO Essential Medicines List and the 4th WHO Essential Medicines List for Children updated in April 2013. (WHO, 2013d) Total medicines in WHO Model List over time is showed in Figure 1-1.

---

[1] Duplicates are defined as molecules that are listed for different indications and are therefore listed many times in different sections of the WHO Model List.

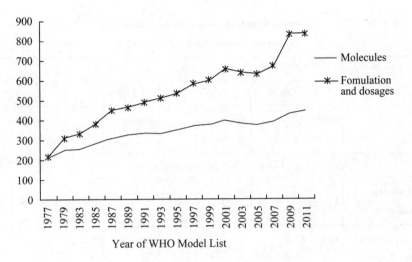

Figure 1-1   Medicines in WHO Model List over time
(including duplicates)(WHO, 2011a)

1.1.4   International progress and achievements

Much has been achieved in pharmaceuticals since the introduction of the essential medicine concept and NEMS. In 1977, only about a dozen countries had what would now be considered an EML or an essential drugs programme. Currently, 160 countries have formal EMLs. More than 90% of the low- and mid-income countries have such lists, while the percentage for high-income countries has reached 60%. (Quick, 2003; WHO, 2004) Over 70 countries have adopted national essential medicine policies. (World Bank, 2010a) The WHO survey of 156 countries in 2007 showed that the number of medicines included in the national EML varies, with a global median of 397, as shown in Table 1-2. The lists are commonly used in public sector procurement across all countries and in high-income countries for public insurance reimbursement. However, only a small fraction of countries use the EML in reimbursement for private insurance. Most of the 130 responding countries (89%) report having a committee for the selection of medicines for national EML. In addition, at least 135 countries have their own therapeutic manuals and formularies, which provide health professionals with current, accurate and unbiased advice on rational use of drugs. (Quick et al., 2002)

Table 1-2   **Details of national essential medicines lists**
by country income level（WHO，2009）

	Country income level*										
	Low(48)		Middle(73)		High(35)		Global(156)	
	yes/resp. countries	% yes	yes/resp. countries	% yes	yes/resp. countries	% yes	yes/resp. countries	% yes
Use of EML in different sectors								
Public sector procurement	44/46	96%	59/65	91%	22/22**	100%	125/133	94%
Public insurance reimbursement**	14/40	35%	20/50**	40%	13/18**	72%	47/108**	44%
Private insurance reimbursement**	4/35	11%	6/49	12%	2/8	25%	12/92**	13%
Committee for EML selection	38/44	86%	59/67	88%	19/19**	100%	116/130	89%
	Median [25%,75%]		Median [25%,75%]		Median [25%,75%]		Median [25%,75%]	
Number of medicines in EML	355 [272, 384] n=34		441 [350, 601] n=52		1706 [1143, 3272] n=8**		397 [334, 580] n=94	

* World Bank List

** More than 30% of countries did not provide an answer to this question.

Furthermore, the concept of essential medicines has also been adopted by many international organizations, including United Nations Children's Fund (UNICEF) and the Office of United Nations High Commissioner for Refugees (UNHCR), as well as by non-governmental organizations and international non-profit supply agencies. Many of these organizations base their medicine supply system on the Model List of WHO.

The essential medicines concept is today a key issue on the international health agenda. Together with the concept of primary health care, it is one of the major achievements of WHO over the last several decades, and its most durable pharmaceutical initiative (Weersuriya & Brudon, 1998). The estimated number of people with access to essential drugs has doubled in only 20 years, from 2.1 billion in 1977 to over 4 billion in 2002. (WHO, 2003b)

1.1.5 Country experiences: three examples

Based on the WHO guideline, countries developed the more specific goals and strategies of NEMS depending upon country situation, national health policy and political priorities set by the government. Here we trace the experiences of three countries as a reference: Tanzania, India and Australia. These three countries have diverse demographic, economic characteristics and health-care financing structures and are in different phases of health technology development.

1.1.5.1 Tanzania

Tanzania is the first country to adopt the essential drugs concept in Africa. The Tanzania Essential Drugs Programme was implemented in 1984, highlighting the government's intention to ensure that qualified effective essential medicines reach all Tanzanians at an affordable price. (WHO, 1993) It also aimed to develop and support national pharmaceutical industries to increase local production and thereby encourage self-reliance. According to Mhamba and Mbirigenda (2010), the existing policy of 1991 contains provisions for :

(1) Drug selection: the policy aims to select pharmaceutical products in accordance with the concept of essential drugs to be distributed as generic drugs;

(2) Procurement: the policy prioritizes essential drugs and preferentially supports local manufacturing companies (who have 15% leeway on prices over international suppliers), and aims to achieve self-reliance by shifting away from imports;

(3) Distribution: essential medicines should always be available to those who need them and should be distributed in the most cost-effective manner;

(4) Quality assurance: facilitated by the Tanzania Food and Drug Authority (TFDA) providing free technical support and regularly inspecting industries; Local industries must register all drugs produced every year after showing that they have achieved GMP.

Information materials such as the Tanzania National Formulary and Standard Treatment Guidelines (STGs) are developed through the programme. The Tanzania EML was last published in 2006, containing over 700 items. This provides minimal protection for local pharmaceutical industries as there are many internationally produced products to choose from. The pharmaceutical sector in Tanzania only consists of eight manufacturing industries all producing generic pharmaceutical products using imported active pharmaceutical ingredients. Tanzania imports about 70% of the national drug requirement and local production accounts for about 30%.

Pharmaceutical products are distributed by the public medical store department (MSD) and 291 TFDA-registered private wholesalers. (Mhamba & Mbirigenda, 2010) The private wholesalers procure from international and local suppliers and distribute to: MSD (through tenders); 352 registered retail pharmacies; 6,000 Duka la Dawas (drug stores licensed to sell only non-prescription medicines) and directly to hospitals. The wholesalers deliver to public health facilities through the MSD public tendering process and to private retail pharmacies and health facilities through direct private procurement processes. The public procurement is done on a competitive basis without any special treatment and/or discrimination against entirely private companies and those in which the government holds 40% shares. (Euro Health Group & MSH-Tanzania, 2007) But Tanzanian bidders enjoy preferential treatment when government issues a tender, and then only need to comply with Tanzanian GMP standards. The MSD runs the tenders and gives a 15% preferential treatment for national suppliers (both local producers and wholesalers).

1.1.5.2　India

India is slow to initiate a comprehensive essential drugs programme, but much has been achieved over the last two decades. In India health is a state subject; national programs for health and medicine pricing are designed by the federal (central) government. The first attempt to introduce essential drugs programme was made in Delhi State, the national capital state of India, in 1994. In 1997 the Delhi Programme was designated INDIA-WHO Essential Drugs Programme by WHO, which was known as Delhi Model. Here we share the specific strategies in Delhi State.

The policy's objective is to improve the availability and accessibility of qualified essential drugs for all those in need. Main contents include: (1) Selection of an EML; (2) Establishment of a pooled procurement system; (3) Preparation of a formulary; (4) Introduction of a quality assurance system; (5) Training in rational prescribing; (6) Provision of drug information (to doctors and for patient guidance); (7) Development of standard treatment guidelines; (8) Research; (9) Monitoring and evaluation; (10) Contents of drug advertising and promotion. The Delhi Society for the Promotion of Rational Use of Drugs (DSPRUD), a non-governmental organization, works in close collaboration with the Delhi Government and with universities to implement various components of the policy. (Chaudhury et al., 2005)

The EML is developed by a committee consisting of a multidisciplinary group of experts using balanced criteria of efficacy, safety, suitability and cost. The first EML was drawn up in 1994 and contained 250 drugs for hospitals and 100 drugs for dispensaries. This is a dynamic list revised every 2 years. In order to provide unbiased information on drugs in the EML, the Essential Drugs Formulary is published, providing the following information for each drug: category of drug, indication, cautions, contraindications, side effects, interactions, dosage forms and dosage. The Delhi STGs are also developed and introduced to prescribers working at dispensaries who are also given a number of training sessions. All the public and private sector doctors in Delhi are given a personal copy of the STGs free of charge. In order to ensure the usage of essential medicines, the expense of non-list medicines should be less than 10% of total medicine expense in general hospitals and 20% in some specific hospitals. (Guan & Shi, 2009)

The procurement of essential medicines is based on competitive bidding through tenders. A Centralized Procurement Agency (CPA) is set up in the Directorate of Health Services to implement the centralized procurement and distribution. The tender process is transparent and there is no preferential buying from state-run units. Pre-qualification of tenders is based on explicit criteria for minimizing the number of tenders, such as GMP, threshold of turnover, manufacturing experiences and et al. The procurement process is called "Two Envelope Selective Tender System"—one with the technical parameters and the other containing the price quotes. The lowest price that qualifies the technical assessment will be selected. The selected manufacturers are required to supply medicines directly to the hospitals or to a central medical store for further distribution to the dispensaries. Basically, the hospitals and other health facilities send their drug requirement to the CPA every 4 months. The CPA places the orders and the manufacturers are required to supply to the health facilities within 35 days.

1.1.5.3　Australia

Australia has emerged as a worldwide leader in drug policy over the last decade, which brought international attention and acclaim. (Norman, 2001) Australia's NEMS was introduced in 2000 and developed collaboratively, with all groups having an interest in medicines in Australia including consumers, health professionals, pharmaceutical industry (including complementary medicines industry), medical media, and state and commonwealth governments. The key policy goals include: timely access to the medicines that Australians need, at a cost individuals and the community can afford; medicines meeting appropriate standards of quality, safety and efficacy; quality use of medicines; and maintaining a responsible and viable medicines industry. (Lofgren & Boer, 2004)

The Pharmaceutical Benefits Schedule (PBS) is part of the NEMS served as an "EML" and provides timely, reliable, and affordable access to necessary medicines for Australians. Drugs listed on the PBS are subsidized by the Australian government for all Australians. The co-payments for medicines are revised annually and currently set at a maximum of AUS $ 34. 20 per item, and AUS $ 5. 60 per item for concession-card holders (aged, disabled, unemployed, etc.). (Yoongthong et al., 2012)

Australia has a well-developed process for the appraisal and listing of drugs and is the first country in the world to introduce cost-effectiveness analysis as a mandatory condition for listing on a national drug formulary. (Hill, Henry & Stevens, 2001) Pharmaceutical Benefits Advisory Committee (PBAC) is an independent statutory committee that meets three times a year to assess applications for listing on the PBS based on the clinical benefit and cost-effectiveness compared with other treatments or products for the same condition.

To ensure the participation in PBS and to encourage prescribing of the most cost-effective agent, the therapeutic group premiums (reference based pricing) are used. The Pharmaceutical Benefits Pricing Authority (PBPA) determines a list of agreed prices which pharmacists (dispensers) pay the pharmaceutical firms for their drugs. The price the government will pay is the lowest for any product in a specific therapeutic group, with the consumer paying any difference to obtain a different product in that group. On the other hand, if the agreed price is above the price paid by consumers, then pharmacists can claim the difference from the government, essentially, consumption of the drug is subsidized. Currently, the PBS has covered more than 2,800 products representing 80% of all dispensed medicines in Australia. (Morgan, McMahon & Greyson, 2008)

1. 1. 5. 4　Summary of implications

The three country stories presented here discussed the country-specific circumstances and factors that shaped their essential medicines programmes with varying degrees of success. There is simply no substitute for that. However, some general, if not universal, implications can still be drawn from their experiences.

The first implication is that, these countries have all involved an emphasis on a list of drugs that embodied the spirit of the essential medicines concept and have evolved to promote rational drug use. The selection of essential medicines is the cornerstone of any essential medicines programme. However, it is crucial to emphasize that the only a list is not enough. The universal access to medicine needs a set of complete policy system to support.

The second implication is that access to essential drugs can be secured only if government plays a strategic role in procuring drugs through a centralized agency such as the CPA in Delhi, or, as in Australia, through subsidizing universal access. Simultaneously, it must institute a system of price control which allows manufacturers and traders modest or reasonable profits. The ability of the procurement agencies to obtain reasonable prices depends upon the size of purchases and their capacity to secure a bargain in the market. Furthermore, the guarantee of reasonable also needs that the cost and value of a medicine are correctly assessed as in Australia on the basis of cost-effectiveness analysis.

The third implication is that health professionals, including physicians, pharmacists and paramedical personnel, have to understand health and pharmaceutical policies. Raising their awareness of rational drug use and essential drugs, and improving their familiarity with products on the market, are therefore urgent tasks. National formularies should be created, suitable for everyday use by practitioners, and be supplied free of charge or at nominal cost. Economic incentives should be used to foster pharmacists' selling of essential drugs.

Lastly, the development of NEMS is dependent on a political commitment on the part of government, an existing basic infrastructure and the support of key stakeholders. National authorities should provide sustained, top-down policy and financial commitment to initiatives fostering a responsible use of medicines.

1. 2 Specific background

1. 2. 1 The history of essential medicines in China

Following the resolution of World Health Assembly, the Chinese government embraced the concept of essential medicines in 1979, but until fairly recently China lacked a comprehensive national policy for essential medicines.

The first edition of national essential medicine list (NEML) in China was produced in 1982, with 278 medicines, all of which were Western medicines (WMs); no traditional Chinese medicines (TCMs) were represented. The list was not updated for ten years because China had no concrete plan to integrate it into healthcare system. In 1991, WHO named China the representative of the Regional Committee for the Western Pacific of the WHO Action Programme on Essential Drugs. This role, along with political considerations, stimulated China's interest in essential medicines. In 1992, a committee which acted as overall managing authority for the selection of essential medicines was assembled. It included representatives from the Chinese Ministry of Health (MoH) and three other government departments. In 1996, the first revised list was issued which increased the number of medicines and included both

Western and Chinese medicines. From then on, the list has been revised every two years. In 2004, it included 2,033 essential medicines for the treatment of most common diseases, with 733 WMs and 1260 TCMs. During this time, the NEML served as a base for the selection of medicine reimbursement lists for social health insurance. (Ye, 2009) From 2004 the NEML ceased updating until the latest NEML was released in 2009. Table 1-3 showed the evolution of NEML in China.

Table 1-3　Number of medicines included in China national essential medicine lists

Edition	1982	1996	1998	2000	2002	2004	2009
WMs	278	699	740	770	759	773	205
TCMs	0	1,699	1,333	1,249	1,242	1,260	102
Total	278	2,398	2,073	2,019	2,001	2,033	307

1.2.2　Essential medicines were not used to their full potential in China

Although the essential medicine list has long existed in China, it has not drawn significant public attention and has never realized its full potential until the most recent health care reform effort. This lack of effectiveness was largely due to China's nascent institutional basis in, and the government's failure to clearly explain, detailed implementation measures for production, distribution, and reimbursement. (Charles & Lu, 2011)

First, the role of essential medicines was weakened with the application of drug reimbursement list under Chinese social health insurance schemes, where drugs are not categorized as essential and nonessential, but as Category A (reimbursable) and Category B (non-reimbursable). (World Bank, 2010a) Thus, "reimbursability" came to overshadow "essentialness".

Second, the fact that hospitals were making profits from reselling medicines also affected the performance of essential medicines. In China the government controlled price schedule for hospitals setting prices for basic health care below cost to keep health care affordable and a 15% profit margin on drugs to make health facilities survive financially. (China NDRC, 2006) However, this price-setting approach induced serious health hazards and physicians tended to over-prescribe, especially the more expensive or profitable medicines, often unnecessary and inappropriate prescriptions. Manufactures and distributors were therefore reluctant to produce the essential medicines that were neither preferred nor profitable. (Chen et al., 2010)

Third, education on the use of new drugs was primarily provided by pharmaceutical distributors and manufacturers' representatives. Disinterested clinical guidelines were not available, especially on the utilization and medical management of essential drugs. It has been fairly easy to promote and reinforce the widespread perception that generic drugs are not as safe, effective, or reliable as brand drugs.

1.2.3   Major problems of China's pharmaceutical sector

Along with the unsuccessful attempts to establish the essential medicine system in China, problems in the pharmaceutical sector have become major sources of public criticism.

In contrast to many countries such as the USA, hospital sectors are the dominant sales channel for pharmaceutical drugs in China, accounting for 70% of all drugs sold and distributed. (Mui & Chee, 2012) Ever since the early 1980s, pharmaceutical revenue has become an overwhelming finance source for most public hospitals, especially at the grassroots level (ranging from 50 to 90 percent of total revenue). This heavy dependence on drug revenues has led to induced consumption and overutilization. As such, the economic impact of the pharmaceutical industry is substantial. Pharmaceutical expenditures have been growing by 15% per year and represented almost 50% of total health spending in China (see Figure 1-2), compared with 18% in countries of the Organization for Economic Co-operation and Development (OECD, 2005). This disparity is partly due to the 15% drug markup policy as mentioned above, which resulted in immense supplier-induced drug expenditures (accounting for 12 to 37 percent of total medical expenditures), and the severity of irrational use of medicines (nearly 80 percent of randomly selected prescriptions were for unnecessary antibiotics). (Charles & Lu, 2011)

In addition, China's pharmaceutical distribution base is extremely fragmented. More than 13,000 pharmaceutical distributors by 2009, and the top three commands only 22% of the market in 2010. Because of this fragmentation, drugs typically flow through several layers of distributors, with multiple handoffs before they reach hospitals or pharmacies. This complex setup means high distribution costs for China. (Mui & Chee, 2012) The commercial promotion activities and profits for multiple layers of distribution contribute a substantial component of the total costs of pharmaceuticals. (Yu, Li, Shi & Yu, 2010)

Basically, the Chinese households devoted 40%-60% of their out-of-pocket health expenditures to medicines. Therefore, the expense of serious family illness, including medicines, is a major financial burden at the household level. Thus, despite the potential health impact of essential medicines, lack of access to essential medicines and irrational medicine use remain serious public health problems in China. These all urge the government to take action.

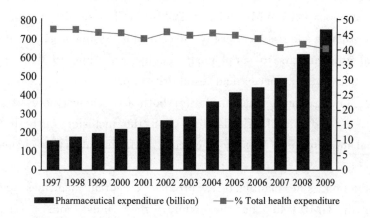

Figure 1-2   Pharmaceutical expenditure in China (1997-2009) [1]

1. 2. 4   The establishment of NEMS under new healthcare reform

In April 2009, the State Council of China released the guidance and plan for a new round of health reform. This 3-year CN¥850 billion ($ 125 billion) reform plan, was the launch of the most radical and comprehensive health reform in Chinese history. (China NDRC, 2009b) It proposed to establish China's NEMS to make essential drugs available, control drug costs and reduce the irrational overuse of drugs, and regarded it as one of five top

---

① Source: China National Health Accounts Report (2010)

priorities in the healthcare reform strategy (2009-2011). (China NDRC, 2009a) It is initially for public primary healthcare facilities, with the intention of extending it to private providers and hospitals.

1.2.4.1　Policy objectives

The objectives of the China's NEMS are: (1) to improve medicine availability, affordability and rational use; and (2) to cut the profit link between health facilities, doctors, and medicines.

1.2.4.2　Policy highlights

The current essential medicine system in China was promulgated with policies and procedures addressing selection, production, procurement, distribution, pricing, utilization and reimbursement.

Selection. The NEML for primary health-care facilities contained 307 generic medicines (205 WMs and 102 TCMs). (Chinese Ministry of Health, 2009) In order to address local need, the central government gave authority to provincial governments to supplement the list according to their economic situation and specific needs and establish a provincial supplemented list (PEML). The appraisal benchmarks for both are: clinical necessity, safety and efficacy, economical affordability, and the inclusion of both Chinese traditional medicine and Western medicine. EML is subject to change every three years.

Production. The manufactures produce essential medicines under the guidance of GMP. In the meanwhile, they must join a centralized pharmaceutical electronic supervision network, attaching a standardized barcode to the smallest package of essential medicines. The essential medicines will be electronically monitored by State Food and Drug Administration (SFDA).

Pricing. The NDRC sets the maximum retail prices of essential medicines, based on which, the actual retail price is determined through competitive bidding by regional authorities.

Procurement and distribution. A province-based centralized procurement system is established. Essential medicines are procured for the whole province in bulk at the agreed bid prices and supplied to facilities for further distribution.

Utilization. Public grass-roots level hospitals may not use any drugs out of EML. Essential medicines are sold for their purchase prices (zero-profit drug policy). Clinic treatment guidelines and formulas for essential medicines are formed. The guidance, covering 18 common diseases encountered in primary care settings, specifies how prescribing physicians should use essential medicines based on a clear diagnosis. The formulary covers 24 treatment categories.

Reimbursement. Local social health insurance programmes must cover all the essential medicines and higher reimbursement is provided for listed drugs than for non-listed drugs.

Generally the National Joint Committee on Essential Drugs (composed of representatives from the nine ministries and coordinated by MoH) will compile the EML and issue policies regarding drug pricing, quality assurance, and compensation of health providers; provincial governments will be in charge of centralized drug tendering and procurement.

1. 2. 4. 3 Strategic significance

The newly-built NEMS goes beyond the scope of an essential medicines list but establishes a "complex system engineering" which is composed of seven interconnected parts. The approach adopted is congruent with the policy spirits expressed by the WHO and could serve as a useful model for other countries in reforming its health care system.

Furthermore, the China's NEMS is highlighted along with four other components of the new healthcare reform: basic medical security, primary health care delivery system, basic public health system, and pilot public hospital reform. Among these five components, essential medicine system is the only reform measure that is related to the transformation of the pharmaceutical sector. The other components of the reform, especially medical institutional reform and medical security reform, could hardly be accomplished if pharmaceutical sector reform is unsuccessful.

Additionally, pharmaceutical sector plays an important role in the medical and health system. Partly due to the distorted health services price schedule and mark-up pricing pattern, which provide incentives for physicians over-providing drugs to patients, pharmaceuticals represent a significant cost driver in health care systems and account for a large share of health expenditures in China (Yu et al., 2010). Therefore, Chinese policy-makers regard the new essential medicine system as a leverage to influence the whole health system.

1. 2. 5　Problem statement

After a program is implemented, even if the program is well organized, efficiently operated, widely utilized, adequately financed, and generally supported by major interest groups, we may still want to ask: Does it work? Do these policies have any beneficial effects on society? Could we do something else with more benefit? Such evaluations are critical to the reform's success and are being encouraged by the government. A policy implementation is exactly viewed as an iterative process in which local experiences are rapidly fed back to policy-makers to revise designs continuously.

Currently, the researches on China's NEMS mainly focused on three aspects. The first kind was referred to theoretical study of policy design and implementation. Before NEMS implementation, most researches emphasized the WHO policy strategies in China's practices, such as Hu et al. (2007) explored the framework of essential medicine system in China from selection, production, circulation, usage, pricing and related finance policies. Shao et al. (2009) particularly discussed the feasible measures related to essential medicines under China's new health reform. After NEMS implementation, the researches turn to focus on the key procedures of current institutional arrangement as well as their logical consequences. For example, Wang and Chen (2010) analyzed the supply and demand mechanism of essential medicines based on the theories of new institutional economics. Liu (2013) discussed the supply chain of essential medicines from a perspective of public governance. The second kind of researches was related to reviews or introductions of international experiences. For example, Sun (2009) reviewed Indian's national policy and analyzed the successful experience of the Delhi Model and hope to make a reference for China, and Wang et al. (2009) systematically reviewed the essential medicine system in seventeen countries and provided decision-making to China's practice. The third kind of researches was referred to empirical studies on implementation process or operational effect. For example, Zhang et al. (2010) analyzed the preliminary effect of zero mark-up policy in community health centers after one-year practice based on the database of Shanghai pharmaceutical purchasing system for hospitals. Li et al. (2011) taking two counties in Shandong province as an sample, compared the changes of prescribing behaviors in township hospitals before and after NEMS.

Generally, the vast bulk came from the first two kinds of researches. A paucity of data existed on empirical studies until 2011. And the prior empirical studies tended to focus on narrow aspects such as the production quality and the selection process for the essential medicines list. It is difficult to make a complete evaluation. Moreover, the method used to analysis was always referred to descriptive analysis of cross-sectional data. The comparative analysis on time-series data or panel data was relatively less. In addition, the previous evaluations were always independent on institutional analysis. The changes of the observed indicators were difficult to attribute to the institutional arrangement. Therefore, there is absolutely a need to explore a method combined policy analysis and empirical investigation, based on full understanding of the characteristics of China's NEMS, to scientifically assess the impact of the new policy.

Given such a background, the present study is put forward and attempts to construct a theoretical framework for assessing NEMS, based on which to develop data collection techniques to obtain empirical evidence thus systematically answering the following questions: What progress has been made? Does it achieve the intended goals? What about the feedback from health-care providers and consumers? What should be done for further advancing the agenda?

1.3   Research goals and objectives

The goal of this study is to explore the implementation and impact of NEMS in China and provide policy implications for the way forward.

The specific objectives include:

(1) To analyze the implementation progress of NEMS across China;

(2) To determine its impact on medicine prices, availability and affordability;

(3) To consider its effect on improving rational drug use;

(4) To explore its impact on the operation of primary health-care facilities;

(5) To investigate the stakeholders' awareness, perception and satisfaction towards NEMS.

1.4 Research methodology and design

This is a pre/post-reform comparative study. The data were selected in 2009 for the pre-reform period and in 2010 and afterwards for post-reform cases.

1.4.1 Data sources

The data were collected by undertaking the desk review, field survey, and focus group discussions and key informant interviews with hospital managers and policy makers.

1.4.1.1 Literature and document review

Domestic and international peer reviewed journals and programs about essential medicines policy to get the knowledge on problem statement, questionnaire and interview form design. Statistic yearbook, national documents from MoH, provincial documents from the local health bureaus were reviewed to gain full understanding of the policy context, approach and implementation progress of NEMS.

1.4.1.2 Field survey

A field survey was used to collect information related to the impact of NEMS, such as drug price information, prescription data, medicine availability information, hospital income and expenditure information and so on. Four provinces (Shandong, Zhejiang, Anhui and Ningxia) were purposively selected as research areas to represent different socio-economic status (SES). Shandong and Zhejiang are located in the Eastern China and have a higher economic level. Anhui is in the Central China and has a middle economic level. Ningxia is in the Western China and has a lower economic level.

The survey in Zhejiang and Anhui was conducted in 2010. It was based on the programme "Mid-term Evaluation on Implementation Effect of Essential Medicines Policy" organized by NDRC. These two provinces are the pioneers in implementing NEMS in China. Two cities in each selected province were chosen by stratified sampling (one with high SES, the other with low). From each of the four selected cities three counties were randomly chosen. All state-own primary health centers (PHCs) in the 12 chosen counties were investigated; the total number was 113.

The survey in Shandong and Ningxia was taken in 2011. A county with a medium size and middle development level in Shandong was selected for sampling. All PHCs in this county were investigated; the total number was 17. In addition, 16 PHCs in Ningxia were selected through stratified sampling. All these counties were already divided by Ningxia local officials into three tiers of SES: high, middle and low. Three counties were randomly selected from the three SES strata; they were Xiji, Tongxin and Qingtongxia. According to the size of the counties, 8 PHCs were randomly selected from Xiji, and 8 PHCs were randomly chosen from the other two selected counties.

1.4.1.3　Focus group discussion and key informant interview

Focus group discussion and key informant interview were used to gain an understanding of stakeholders' perceptions on NEMS and their views on its impact, and to provide supplementary information for quantitative investigations. A group of health bureau officials, hospital managers as well as department heads in each county were organized for discussions and interviews.

1.4.2　Data collection

Data were collected by trained university students and supervised by the survey manager and the principal investigator.

Three self-compiled questionnaires were used for the field survey in all sample PHCs. The first is to survey the basic information of PHC and items include hospital size, number of patients, hospital income and expenditure and so on (see Appendix I). The second is for medicine prices survey and items include medicine name, dosage, form, price and sales (see Appendix II). The third is used in survey on social satisfaction. It has two versions: one is for rural residents (see Appendix III) and the other is for primary health workers (Appendix IV).

The prescriptions for outpatients were selected using systematic random sampling in each PHC. Data collection was anonymous (name or identifying information of the patients, general practitioners, and pharmacists were not obtained).

Semi-structured question sheet was prepared in key informant interviews and focus group discussions. Questions included the features of local practice，the impact of NEMS on health utilization，the encountered challenges and the suggestions for further improvement (see Appendix V).

1.4.3　Data analysis

Data from questionnaire survey and documents review were used to quantitatively assess the effect of NEMS on policy objectives. For supplementing the quantitative analysis，data from the interviews and focus group discussions was transcribed and analyzed in relation to the themes studied. The detailed analysis method was described in the following chapter.

1.4.4　Data quality assurance

The completeness, consistency and clarity of data are assured by quality control mechanisms throughout all phases of data collection, entry, and analysis.

Prior to data collection，the principal investigator had contacted the hospital directors in order to ensure good cooperation between hospital staff and the team of researchers. All data collectors were well trained in data collection skills and ethical approach，including confidentiality. During field survey，data collectors clearly explained the purpose of investigations. Completed questionnaires were checked on the spot. Any missing questions and errors were corrected by returning to the respondents when possible. The key researchers conducted the interviews and mediated the focus group discussions. Daily meetings of the research team were assured during the data collection. Whole questions encountered were discussed and experiences of each investigator were exchanged，including how to relax the participants，how to make respondents understand questions easily，how to better organize interviews and reduce disturbances. During the data entry，a double-checked was used. The questionnaire where a discrepancy found and cannot be corrected was excluded.

1.5　Potential contributions

This study provides a framework for assessing NEMS based on which to investigate its effect on improving access to and rational use of medicines in rural China and identify promising ideas for the way forward. Its major contributions can be summarized as follows.

Firstly, this study provides a comprehensive description of the large-scale essential medicines reform under way in China. To the authors' knowledge, no prior detailed description of activities under this reform component has been published previously.

Secondly, an effective tool is put forward to assess and monitor NEMS. It contains a comprehensive set of simple and reliable indicators which can be adapted to fit national contexts. The survey method for these indicators is based on the recommendation of the WHO and its partners. This tool allows regions and countries to monitor the processes by which a national drug policy is implemented and the changes over a period of time. The detailed method has been described and is easily replicable.

Thirdly, the study also develops a simplified hospital operation model and provides insight on policy adjustments about hospital compensation followed with the introduction of NEMS. This model quantitatively simulates the structure and behaviors of the real system related to hospital income and expenditure and might be broadened to a simulated platform for policy research.

Fourthly, this study enriches the current monitoring and evaluation research on NEMS. It serves as a reference in terms of research approach and contents for policy makers and government organizations and recommendations could be incorporated into the national medicine policy. To some extent, the results of this work might be also useful to international agencies, such as the WHO, and governments of developing nations in advocating for the incorporation of NEMS. Furthermore, it creates a new standard by which comparisons can be made between areas, between countries or over time.

1. 6 Design and organization

Part I of this book consists of 8 sections as follows:

Chapter 1 describes the general and specific background, which corresponds to the international and domestic rationality about essential medicines. Also, the research goals and objectives, potential contributions and statement of originality are listed in this section, accompanied by research methodology and organization.

Chapter 2 presents the theoretical and methodological consideration for the proposed policy evaluation of NEMS based on the literature review.

Chapter 3 analyzes the progress and challenges on the implementation of China's NEMS, especially in the four studied provinces. It provides a policy base for the impact evaluation in the following chapters.

Chapter 4 measures the price changes of essential medicines in rural China before and after the implementation of NEMS and provides updated data on how people pay for medicines and how prices change with time, thereby evaluates the impact of NEMS on medicine access.

Chapter 5 investigates the outcome of the NEMS objectives in terms of rational drug use in rural primary health centers and provides quantitative information for monitoring and improving prescribing process in grassroots level hospitals.

Chapter 6 evaluates the impact of NEMS using facilities as the basis of the analysis, and mainly focuses on the medicines availability and hospital financial operation. Also, it explores the feasible measures of hospital compensation for the NEMS-related reductions based on Dynamic Synthesis Methodology.

Chapter 7 explores the awareness, perception and satisfaction with respect to NEMS among the residents and professionals and to provide the baseline data for policy improvement.

The last section is the conclusion and it puts forward the policy recommendations for improving NEMS. Also, the limitations of the current study are discussed and the perspectives for future work are illustrated.

Chapter 2   Theoretical and methodological consideration

This chapter presents theoretical and methodological consideration for the proposed policy evaluation based on literature review. First, it illustrates a theoretical and conceptual framework of China's NEMS and then some common models of policy evaluation. Next, following the introduction of the existing monitoring tools for pharmaceutical situations, a two-level indicator-based monitoring strategy is developed and used to monitor NEMS in this research. All these provides the framework for field survey design and data collection. The final model of System Dynamics introduced in this chapter was used in chapter 6 for policy simulation, following the preliminary analysis of data.

2. 1   Definition of items

2. 1. 1   Access to medicines

The indicator on "Access to Medicines (ATM)" was created by the WHO in the mid-1990s and has been used since then. Medicines access is defined as the equitable availability and affordability of essential medicines during the process of medicine acquisition. (WHO, 2003c) In this definition, physical availability is a basic measure of ATM. It means that essential medicines to treat common diseases should be available in all facilities, especially in public sector facilities. To measure affordability of basic pharmaceutical treatment is as another indicator of ATM. Affordability is expressed as the ratio of the cost of treating a moderate condition to a standard unit of measure. Countries may identify an optional unit of measure (e.g. poverty line, basket of food, the lowest daily government salary and so on). Universal medicine access has been included in the objectives of the Millennium Development. (WHO, 2004b)

2.1.2 Rational use of medicines

The rational drug use (RDU) is defined as "patients receive medications appropriate to their clinical needs, in doses that meet their own individual requirements, for an adequate period of time, and at the lowest cost to them and their community" (WHO, 2004a). Irrational use occurs when one or more of these conditions are not met. Examples of irrational use of medicines include: use of too many medicines per patient (poly-pharmacy); inappropriate use of antimicrobials, often in inadequate dosage, for non-bacterial infections; over-use of injections when oral formulations would be more appropriate; failure to prescribe in accordance with clinical guidelines; inappropriate self-medication, often of prescription-only medicines; non-adherence to dosing regimens. (WHO, 2012a)

2.1.3 Primary health centers

In China, the primary health center (PHC) is the basic structural and functional unit of the health services and often referred to as the grassroots level hospital. It is established to provide accessible, affordable and available primary health care to people.

2.1.4 Essential medicines

Essential medicines include national essential drugs (NEDs) and provincial supplement essential drugs (PEDs) in China. Furthermore, throughout this study, the words "drug" "medicine" and "pharmaceutical" are used interchangeably.

2.2 Program logic model of China's NEMS

Evaluating a program entails understanding how the program operates and what it is intended to accomplish. Program logic models are visual representations of programs showing how a program is intended to work; that is, how resources that are available to deliver the program are converted into program activities, and how those activities in turn produce intended results. (McDavid & Hawthorn, 2006) The logic model is a theoretical framework of a program, including the components, policy outputs and outcomes. Policy components are clusters of activities in the program. Policy outputs are typical ways of representing the amount of work that is done as policy is implemented. Each component is connected to the specific outputs. Policy outcomes are the intended results that are linked to policy objectives.

The central government guidance on NEMS has depicted a clear picture of the implementation process. As planned, the new system would flow linearly from definition of the EML, production and tendering for drugs on the list, distribution, delivery and use of essential drugs. The ultimate purpose is to deliver safe, effective, and affordable drugs to local communities, promote rational drug use, lower drug costs and improve health status of the people.

So in this case, the components of NEMS are selection, production, pricing, procurement, distribution, utilization, and reimbursement. Policy outputs include: development of EML; production under the guidance of GMP; centralized pharmaceutical electronic supervision network; setting price ceilings of essential medicines; province-based competitive bidding and centralized procurement; zero-profit medicine policy; stock only essential medicines and mandatory use; development of clinic treatment guidelines and formulas for essential medicines; and expanded coverage and increased reimbursement rate of social health insurance. The outcomes are expected to be ATM (affordability and availability) and RDU.

Figure 2-1 illustrates the logic model of China's NEMS. Within this framework, price ceiling could avoid the failure of price mechanism; the centralized procurement could strengthen the market competition and simplify the supply chain, which is effective to reduce prices for essential medicines. Consumers have greater protection through quality standards and more confidence in the quality of medicines. State-run primary health settings may not use any drugs out of EML. Essential medicines should be sold at the procurement prices and the distorted revenue-generating mechanism of the hospital could be abandoned, thus reducing the incentives for over-prescription. The joint regulation of EML，clinic treatment guidelines and formulas for essential medicines would increase the knowledge of rational medicines use and improve prescribing behaviors.

Therefore，view from the top-level design，the implementation of NEMS can achieve the stated policy objectives in theory. What we do in this study is to assess whether and at what extent NEMS can achieve the intended objectives in the reality.

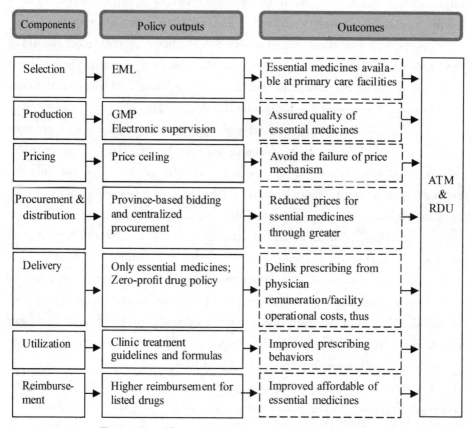

Figure 2-1　The program logic model of China NEMS

2. 3　Theory and method of policy evaluation

2. 3. 1　The concept of policy evaluation

Policy evaluation is concerned with learning about the consequences of public policy. It means evaluating alternative public policies as contrasted with describing them or explaining why they exist. (Lester & Stewart, 2000) Essentially, there are two distinctive tasks in policy evaluation. One task is to determine what the consequences of a policy are by describing its impact, and the other task is to judge the success or failure of a policy according to a set of standards or value criteria. (Dubnick & Bardes, 1983)

One of the key questions that many policy evaluations are expected to address can be worded as follows: To what extent, if any, did the policy/program achieve its intended objectives? Usually, we assume that the policy in question is "aimed" at some intended objective(s). Figure 2-2 offers a picture of this expectation. The arrow connecting the policy/program and its intended objective(s) is a key part of most program evaluations. It shows that the policy/program is intended to cause the outcomes. And the "?" above the arrow now raises the key question of whether the program caused the outcomes.

The main intended outcomes of China's NEMS are ATM and RDU as summarized above. Thus, with respect to the evaluation of NEMS in this study, the key question is: to what extent, dose NEMS improve medicines' access and rational use?

Figure 2-2　The concept of policy evaluation

2. 3. 2　Common evaluation models

Program evaluation involves comparisons designed to estimate what changes in society can be attributed to the program. Ideally, this means comparing what "actually happened" to "what would have happened if the program had never been implemented". It is not difficult to measure what happened; the real problem is to measure what would have happened without a program and then compare the two conditions of society. (Dye, 2010) There are several common research designs in policy evaluation.

2.3.2.1　Before versus After Comparisons

The before and after study is the most common way of comparison, which compares results in a jurisdiction at two times—one before the program is implemented and the other after it is implemented. Usually only target groups are examined. These before and after comparisons are designed to show program impacts, but it is very difficult to know whether the changes observed, if any, came about as a result of the program or as a result of other changes that were occurring in society at the same time. (see Design 1, Figure 2-3)

2.3.2.2　Projected Trend Line versus Postprogram Comparisons

A better estimation of what would have happened without the program can be made by projecting past (preprogram) trends into the postprogram time period. Then these projections can be compared with what actually happened in society after the program was implemented. The differences between the projections based on preprogram trend and the actual postprogram data can be attributed to the program itself. Note that data on target groups or conditions must be obtained for several periods before the program was initiated, so that a trend line can be established (see Design 2, Figure 2-3). This design is better than the before and after design, but it requires more efforts by program evaluators.

2.3.2.3　Comparisons between Jurisdictions with and without Programs

Another common evaluation design is to compare individuals who have participated in programs with those who have not, or to compare cites, states, or nations which have programs with those that do not. Comparisons are sometimes made in the postprogram period only. But so many other differences exist between individuals or jurisdictions that it is easy to attribute differences in their conditions to differences in policy programs. Some of the problems involved can be resolved if we observe both kinds of jurisdictions before and after the introduction of the program. This enables to estimate differences between jurisdictions before program efforts are considered. After the program is initiated, we can observe whether the differences between jurisdictions have widened or not (see Design 3, Figure 2-3).

2.3.2.4　Comparisons between Control and Experimental Groups before and after Program Implementation

This research design involves the careful selection of control and experimental groups that are identical in every way, the application of the policy to the experimental group only, and the comparison of changes in the experimental group with changes in the control group after the application of the policy. Initially, control and experimental groups must be identical, and the preprogram performance of each group must be measured and found to be the same. The program must be applied only to the experimental group. The postprogram differences between the experimental and control groups must be carefully measured. (see Design 4, Figure 2-3)

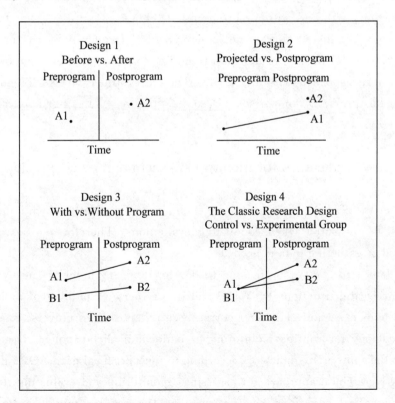

Figure 2-3　Common research designs in program evaluation (Dye, 2010)

2.3.2.5 The option in this study

Basically, each research design has its own advantages and disadvantages. The final option should be based on the actual condition of the program. This study chose the research design of before versus after Comparison. Firstly, The NEMS is implemented based on county/city pilot. The condition can be deemed homogeneous in one pilot site. However the primary health facilities in the same county are implemented nearly at the same time. It is impossible to split them into control and experimental groups. Therefore, Comparison between Control and Experimental Groups before and after Program Implementation (Design 4, Figure 2-3) is not applicable in this study. Secondly, there are many differences between jurisdictions, such as the economic development level and the population size. It is easy to attribute differences in their conditions to differences in the implementation of NEMS, thereby influencing the judgment. Therefore, Comparison between Jurisdictions with and without Programs (Design 3, Figure 2-3) is also not applicable. Thirdly, China's drug policy changed frequently in the previous years, so it is difficult to establish a trend line for a better estimation of what would have happened without NEMS. Therefore, the Projected Trend Line versus Postprogram Comparison (Design 2, Figure 2-3) is not applicable in this study.

2.4 Indicators for monitoring essential medicine policy

For the research design, it is necessary to know exactly which indicators should be measured when conducting evaluations. Therefore, a systematic method of gathering data is needed.

Many efforts have been done to develop tools to monitor and evaluate pharmaceutical situations by WHO and its partners. A number of indicator-based tools exist now. However currently, there is still no universally agreed methodology for routine monitoring of national medicine policy. Users can select the appropriate indicators according to their practical needs. Overall, the WHO hierarchical approach for assessing, monitoring and evaluating country pharmaceutical situations has proven that the regular monitoring is not difficult and can be done in a cost-efficient manner compared with others.

(WHO, 2007b) The WHO/HAI measurement method is identified as a validated and internationally accepted means of collecting reliable evidence on medicine prices and availability. (WHO, 2012b) More than 60 national surveys have been done under the guidance of this manual. The best way to investigate drug use in health facilities is by the usage of indicators created and validated by the WHO/INRUD, which have been used extensively in many countries. (World Health Organization, 1993) These three methodologies have been summarized as below in order to provide references for developing a practical monitoring strategy for national essential medicine policy.

2. 4. 1 WHO hierarchical approach

The WHO hierarchical approach is built around three groups of core indicators: Level I, Level II and Level III (see Figure 2-4). (WHO, 2007b) These core indicators systematically measure the most important information needed to gain a comprehensive picture of the pharmaceutical situation in a country. Level I indicators provide a rapid means of obtaining information on the existing infrastructure and key processes of national pharmaceutical system. The indicators are assessed by a short questionnaire completed at national level. The results provide a range of descriptions of existing structures and processes, and can illustrate the country's capacity to implement policy in specific areas of the pharmaceutical sector. Level II indicators provide systematic data to measure outcomes on the access and rational use of medicines. Data on these indicators are collected through facility-based surveys. The results of surveys can be used to indicate the extent to which the objectives set by the pharmaceutical sector have been achieved. Level III indicators are a more detailed list of indicators covering key components and areas such as medicine pricing, medicine supply management, HIV/AIDS, TRIPS, and regulatory capacity assessment.

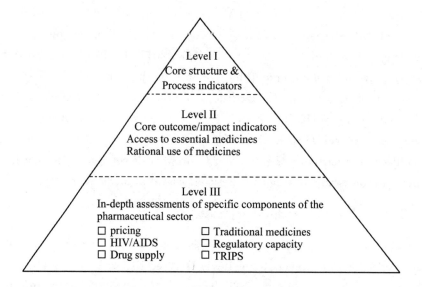

Figure 2-4   Levels of core indicators in WHO hierarchical approach (WHO, 2007b)

The pharmaceutical components in Level I indicators include: written implementation plan about national medicines policy, regulatory system, medicine supply system, medicine financing, production and trade and rational use system (such as standard treatment guidelines, curricula and continuing education programmes, medicine information centers and public education campaigns). The Level II facility core outcome indicators support the Level I structure and process indicators by providing specific data about important pharmaceutical outcomes. These indicators which have been summarized in Table 2-1 measure the degree of attainment of strategic pharmaceutical objectives.

Table 2-1   The Level II facility core outcome indicators in

WHO hierarchical approach (WHO, 2007b)

Access

Availability of key medicines in public health facility dispensaries, private drug outlets and warehouses supplying the public sector

Percentage of Prescribed medicines dispensed or administered to patients at public health facility dispensaries

Average stockout duration in public health facility dispensaries and warehouses supplying the public sector

Adequate record in public health facility dispensaries and warehouses supplying the public sector

Affordability of treatment for adults and children under 5 years of age at public health facility dispensaries and private drug outlets

Price of key medicines in public health facility dispensaries and private drug outlets

Price of pediatric medicines in public health facility dispensaries and private drug outlets

Average cost of medicines at public health facilities and private drug outlets

Geographical accessibility of public health facility dispensaries and private drug outlets

Quality

Percentage of medicines expired in public health facility dispensaries, private drug outlets and warehouses supplying the public sector

Adequacy of conservation conditions and handling of medicines in public health facility dispensaries and warehouses supplying the public sector

Rational use of medicines

Percentage of medicines adequately labeled at public health facility dispensaries and private drug outlets

Percentage of patients knowing how to take medicines at public health facility dispensaries and private drug outlets

Average number of medicines per prescription at public health facility dispensaries and public health facilities

Percentage of patients prescribed antibiotics in public health facilities

Percentage of patients prescribed injections in public health facilities

Percentage of prescribed medicines on the essential medicines list at public health facilities

Percentage of medicines prescribed by generic name at public health facilities

Availability of standard treatment guidelines at public health facilities

Availability of essential medicine list at public health facilities

Percentage of tracer cases treated according to the recommended treatment protocol/guide at public health facilities

Percentage of prescription medicines bought with no prescription

Continued

Other information

Percentage of of facilities that comply with the law（presence of a pharmacist）
Percentage of facilities with pharmacist, nurse, pharmacy aide/health assistant or untrained staff dispensing
Percentage of facilities with doctor, nurse, trained health worker/health aide prescribing
Percentage of facilities with prescriber trained in RDU

2.4.2　WHO/HAI measurement method

The WHO/HAI Project on medicine prices, availability and affordability, established in 2001, is a collaborative partnership between WHO and the international non-governmental organization Health Action International. （WHO/HAI, 2003） The project's objective is to develop a reliable methodology for collecting and analyzing medicine price, availability, affordability and medicine price component data across health-care sectors and regions in a country and to improve access to essential medicines. （WHO/HAI, 2008） This approach is designed to measure medicine prices and availability at a certain point in time, but can also be used to monitor them over a period of time. It is characterized as follows: 1) standard global and regional lists of medicines for international comparisons; 2) use of international reference prices; 3) comparison of originator brand and generically equivalent medicines; 4) sector comparisons: public, private and other sectors; 5) treatment affordability comparisons; 6) identification of price components, e.g. taxes and mark-ups.

In order to make the survey manageable and to ensure comparability, a short core list of medicines has been selected as the basis for data collection and analysis. The global core list contains 14 medicines and each regional core list contains additional 16 medicines, respectively. For each medicine, the core list contains one dosage form, one strength and one recommended pack size. The 30 medicines contained in the core list are selected to indicate a range of treatments for common acute and chronic conditions that cause substantial morbidity and mortality. They are recommended, usually as first-line courses of treatment, in global, regional, and national treatment guidelines and most are included in the WHO Model List of Essential Medicines.

As for the outcome measurement, the availability of individual medicines is reported as the percentage of medicine outlets where an individual medicine product is found. Bear in mind that the availability data only refers to the day of data collection and may not reflect the average monthly or yearly availability of medicines at individual facilities. Medicine prices are expressed as ratios relative to a standard set of international reference prices (IRPs), known as the median price ratio (MPR). The ratio is an expression of how much greater or less the local medicine price is than the international reference price, e.g. an MPR of two would mean that the local medicine price is twice that of the IRP. The Management Sciences for Health (MSH) provides the reference prices, which are offered by mostly not-for-profit suppliers to developing countries for multi-source products. (MSH, 2009) The affordability of treating key health problems using standardized treatment regimens is calculated using the median prices collected during the survey. The treatment cost is compared to the daily wage of the lowest-paid unskilled government worker to determine the number of days' wages needed to pay for the cost of treatment.

2.4.3　WHO/INRUD manual for drug use

In 1989, the International Network for the Rational Use of Drugs (INRUD) was formed to conduct multi-disciplinary intervention research projects to promote more rational use of medicines. (WHO, 2002c). Following this, a WHO/INRUD manual was developed for investigating drug use in primary health care facilities. (WHO, 1993b). This manual sets out a simple and reliable methodology for gathering essential data on drug use patterns and prescribing behavior in health facilities. A brief list of the core drug use indicators is presented in Table 2-2. This methodology, which has been widely tested in a number of developing countries, is proved both feasible to measure and informative as first-level indicators.

Table 2-2　　　　**WHO/INRUD drug use indicators for primary
health-care facilities**（WHO，1993b）

Prescribing indicators
Average number of medicines prescribed per patient encounter
Percentage of medicines prescribed by generic name
Percentage of encounters with an antibiotic prescribed
Percentage of encounters with an injection prescribed
Percentage of medicines prescribed from essential medicine list or formulary
Patient care indicators
Average consultation time
Average dispensing time
Percentage of medicines actually dispensed
Percentage of medicines adequately labeled
Percentage of patients with knowledge of correct doses
Facility indicators
Availability of essential medicine list or formulary to practitioners
Availability of key medicines

The drug use indicators are typically measured with a defined geographic or administrative area, either to describe drug use at a given point in time or to monitor changes over time. All of the data needed to measure the core indicators are collected from medical records or direct observations at individual health facilities. The values of drug-use indicators can be used to assess the problems of clinically or economically inappropriate drug use, to make comparisons between groups or to measure changes over time, as a supervisory tool to identify individual prescribers or health facilities with especially poor patterns of drug use, and to measure the effect of interventions.

Table 2-3 lists reference values for some prescribing indicators derived from WHO documents and literatures. In this study, the medication is recognized more reasonable if the observed value of RDU indicators is closer to the ideal value.

Table 2-3 **Derived reference values for WHO prescribing indicators**

Indicators	Ideal value	WHO standard value (1997)	Observed value in 11 developing countries (1993)	Observed value in 35 countries (2004)	Observed values in WHO monitoring (2006)	
					Median (25%,75%) of 57 low-income countries	Median (25%,75%) of 65 middle-income countries
No. of drug per prescription	<2	1.6-1.8	1.3-3.8	2.39	2.7(2.2-2.9)	2.5(2.4-3.0)
Percentage of antibiotics	<30.0	20.0-26.8	27-63	44.8	51.7(45.0-60.0)	43.3(36.7-50.0)
Percentage of injection	<20.0	13.4-24.1	0.2-48	22.8	23.1(11.3-28.8)	6.7(0-10.5)
Percentage of generics	100.0	100.0	37-94			
Percentage of EMs	100.0	100.0	86-88			
Consultation time (min)			2.3-6.3			
Dispensing time (sec)			12.5-86.1			
Percentage of knowledge of dosage			27-82			
Percentage of drugs dispensed			70-83			
Percentage of drugs in stock			38-90			
Percentage of impartial information			40			

2.4.4 Indicator-based monitoring strategy for China's NEMS

Based on the international experiences and China national conditions, an indicator-based monitoring strategy is developed in this study for China's NEMS, as shown in Table 2-4. The monitoring strategy follows the concept of WHO hierarchical approach and consists of two-level indicators: core structure and process indicators (Level I) and core outcome/impact indicators (Level II).

Table 2-4   Indicator-based monitoring strategy for China's NEMS

Level I Core structure and process indicators	EML formulation
	Centralized procurement system
	Distribution and delivery system
	Medicine financing
	Compensation mechanism
Level II Core outcome/impact indicators	Access
	Medicine prices and affordability
	Availability of essential medicines in hospital
	Rational use
	Average number of drugs prescribed per encounter
	Percentage of drugs prescribed from national EML
	Average number of antibiotics prescribed per encounter
	Percentage of encounters with an antibiotic prescribed
	Percentage of encounters with an injection prescribed
	Percentage of encounters with hormone prescribed
	Average medicine cost per encounter

The core structure and process indicators are concerned with key components of China's NEMS, centering on formulation of EML, centralized procurement system, distribution and delivery system, medicine financing and compensation mechanism for primary health-care facilities. The information is mainly collected through desk review. The results could provide a range of descriptions of existing structures and processes, and can illustrate the progress in implementation of China's NEMS.

The selection of core outcome/impact indicators is derived from WHO/ HAI method and WHO/INRUD method. ATM is observed in terms of availability and affordability and RDU is measured from prescribing behaviors and prescription cost. Data used to measure these indicators is collected through facility-based survey. The findings could elegantly answer whether people have access to essential medicines and whether these medicines are being properly used. However, the measurement method is not completely replicated. NEMS is important for public primary health settings. Little information can be obtained with respect to private sectors and other outlets. Therefore, the core outcome indicators are typically measured within public primary sectors. Additionally, we give up the measurement of patient care indicators exactly due to the difficulty of acquiring the indicator values before NMES for comparison.

2.5 Fieldwork design

A field survey is designed to collect core outcome/impact information in this research. In addition to the intended policy objectives, the spillover effects of NEMS should be considered as well. The most obvious is the survival crisis of primary health-care facilities due to the medicine zero-profit policy, because more than 50% of their operating budget is from the drug sales. Furthermore, the public feedback should be another factor to consider. They are the main stakeholders of the healthcare reform. Therefore, we expand the concept of policy evaluation in this study and focus not only on its intended objectives but also on the spillover effects as well as the social feedbacks. Figure 2-5 depicts a picture of the fieldwork design.

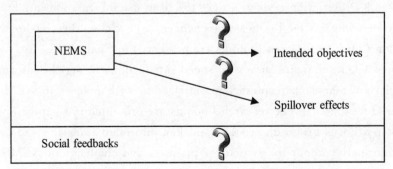

Figure 2-5　The fieldwork design for evaluation of NEMS

2.5.1 Survey objectives

The survey is aimed to collect information related to the impact of NEMS. It is designed to measure the outcomes in 2010 and 2011, and then make a comparison with 2009. In consequence, the survey enables the following questions to be answered:

(1) Are the essential medicines being available in primary health centers?

(2) What price do people pay for these medicines?

(3) Are these medicines being used properly?

(4) What about the operation of primary health centers under NEMS?

(5) Are the public satisfied with the NEMS?

2.5.2 Steps in the survey

Data collection takes place according to the following five steps and the details will be described in the subsequent chapters. Sampling is done to ensure the findings are representative in China. Information about questionnaires can be found on appendices.

Step 1 Questionnaire survey on the operation of PHC: to get the information on medical service, medicines availability, income & expenditure information, and so on. These data can be used to answer Questions (1) and (4) and the key research findings are presented in Chapter 6.

Step 2 Questionnaire survey on medicine prices: to get the information of medicine prices in 2009-2011. These data can be used to answer Question (2) and make comparisons to measure changes over time. The research findings are presented in Chapter 4.

Step 3 Prescription review: to get the drug use information in 2009-2011 and make comparisons to measure changes over time, thereby answering Question (3). The research findings are presented in Chapter 5.

Step 4 Questionnaire survey on social satisfaction: to get the information on social awareness, perception and satisfaction with respect to NEMS and answer Question (5). The research findings are presented in Chapter 7.

Step 5 Focus group discussions and key informant interview: to get the local information about the structure, process, and challenge of NEMS. Key findings are presented in Chapter 3.

2. 6   Other methods used in this research

Health care system is complex. It showed both detailed complexity (large number of elements) and dynamic complexity (many interconnections). Systems approach is proved to be an effective way to deal with this complexity. In the spectrum of systems approaches, system dynamics (SD) is among the most quantitative and analytical and is problem-focused and policy-oriented. SD is to build models of a real world and to study how its (real world's) structure produces dynamic behavior over time (J. Sterman, 2000). Originally developed in the 1950s to help corporate managers improve their understanding of industrial processes, SD is currently being used throughout the public and private sectors for policy analysis and design. In the health field, studies can go back more than 30 years and include a variety of studies of health care delivery and epidemiology. (Marna, Jack & William, 2005)

SD applications involve the development of causal diagrams and computer simulation models that are unique to each problem setting. The causal loop diagram, as depicted in Figure 2-6 (a), is a simple map of a system with all its components and their cause and effect relationships. The creation of causal loop diagrams is the qualitative part of the SD methodology, which forms the hypothesized dynamic structure of the system. A cause and effect relationship can change the behavior in the same direction (indicated with a plus sign) or in the opposite direction (indicated with a minus sign). To perform a more detailed quantitative analysis, a causal loop diagram is needed to transform to a stock and flow diagram as illustrated in Figure 2-6 (b). A stock and flow model helps to study and analyze the system in a quantitative way. Stock variables (rectangles) represent the state variables and are the accumulations in the system and also called level variables. Flow variables (valves) alter the stocks by filling or draining the stocks and the rate of change. A flow is the rate of change in a stock. So the flow variable is also called rate variables. Arrows point to the causal relation between two variables and also reflect the flow of information within the model structure.

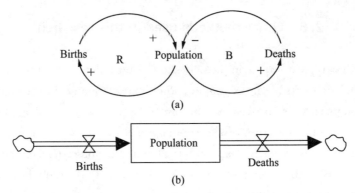

Figure 2-6　Causal loops diagram（a）and stock and flow diagram（b）

The development of a computer simulation model is based upon a stock and flow diagram and equations which depict interrelated variables in the system. The interlocking set of differential and algebraic equations in a SD model is always developed from a broad spectrum of relevant measured and experiential data. A completed model may contain scores or hundreds of equations along with the appropriate numerical inputs. (Sterman, 2000) Such SD models can be used for "what-if" questions to experiment with alternative scenarios by changing the values of the variables in the model. The output of the simulation can then be compared with that of the real world.

Thus, an SD analysis involves the following five steps: (1) Problem articulation; (2) Formulation of dynamic hypothesis; (3) Formulation of a simulation model; (4) Testing; (5) Policy design and evaluation. (Goh & Love, 2012) Problem articulation involves specifying the problem of concern. The formulation of dynamic hypothesis usually employs qualitative methods to create causal loop diagrams. Simulation model is assessed for their ability to imitate actual trends that have been observed in the real world. Other tests that can be undertaken include extreme condition tests to ensure that robustness of model against extreme values in key variables, and sensitivity analyses to determine the impact of uncertainties on model outputs. Once a model is deemed to be credible it can be used for policy analysis, where users can assess a range of policy options by modifying different variables for specific time periods.

Chapter 3 Current progress on the implementation of China's NEMS

Under the broad direction of NEMS, many localities experiment with innovative ways to improve their own local systems. This chapter analyzes the implementation progress of NEMS across China, especially in the four studied provinces, based on document review and key informant interview. It provides a policy foundation for the impact evaluation in the following chapters.

3. 1 Overall progress in implementation

In 2009, right after the announcement of the new national health care reform plan, the government issued the "Implementation Plan of Essential Medicine System in China," "Management of Essential Medicine Formulary (Temporary)," and "Essential Medicine Formulary for Grassroots Health Care Institutions" successively to guide the implementation of essential medicine system. In addition, health authorities set up a buffer period for primary health-care facilities to use up or dispose of all non-essential drugs, usually 2 to 3 months. But during the buffer period, all non-essential drugs should be sold at cost. By July 2011, all 31 provinces have adopted the NEML and the province-based centralized procurement system as well as the zero-profit policy for public primary health-care facilities. (Chinese MoH, 2011b) Most provinces have formulated the supplementary PEML.

3.2 Essential medicine list

3.2.1 National essential medicine list

The NEML includes 307 medicines comprising 205 chemical medicines covering 24 categories of diseases and 102 TCMs covering six categories of clinical indications. A large proportion of the medicines can be used to treat diseases with high prevalence in China.

By comparing the WHO model list and the China's NEML, we can see some important differences (see Table 3-1). First, the quantity of included Western medicines varies substantially. As a result, the diseases covered by the two lists are different. The WHO list covers some important diseases such as cancers that China's list does not cover. Second, medicine classification varies between them. The Anatomical Therapeutic Chemical Classification is used in the WHO list to classify medicines while Clinical Pharmacology Classification is used for Western medicines in China's list. This is because the NEML may need to conform to other medicine lists for social health insurance schemes. (Wang & Zhang, 2011) Third, the WHO has selected essential medicines for children. Even though a group of national representatives in China urge the government to take actions for children, no official response has been found for this appeal yet.

Table 3-1   Discrepancies between the WHO model list and China's NEML

Items	WHO model list (the 17th edition)	China's NEML
Medicines	358	357
WMs	358	255
TCMs	0	102
Complementary medicines	Complementary list	Provincial selection
Revising interval	2 years	3 years
Classification method	Anatomical Therapeutic Chemical Classification	Clinical Pharmacology Classification

Continued

Defined forms for Western medicines	Yes	Yes
Supporting documents	STGs, formulary for essential medicines	National formulary and guideline for EMs
EML for children	Yes	No

3. 2. 2　Provincial lists of supplemented medicines

By May 2012, all 31 provinces had published their own lists with additional WMs and TCMs based on NEML except Tibet. Tibet published provincial list only with additional 455 Tibetan medicines. Shandong province and Jilin province have published separate lists for urban and rural areas. In terms of the number of medicines selected, the provincial selection (except Tibet) ranges between 64 and 381 with an average of 215. Shanghai's expansion was the largest whereas Ningxia added only 64. Table 3-2 presents the quantity of medicines in PEMLs of the four studied provinces. A survey finds that more developed provinces include more medicines than less developed provinces (see Figure 3-1). (Wang & Zhang, 2011) Additionally, the quantity of WMs is more than TCMs in most PEMLs. The proportion of TCMs in PEMLs is about 14. 12%-57. 81%, with an average of 38. 73%. The supplemented medicines cover all the categories found in the NEML as well as a new category for antineoplastic medicines.

Table 3-2　　Quantity of medicines in provincial supplement lists of the four studied provinces

Provinces	Selected medicines	Selected western medicines		Selected TCMs	
	N	N	%	N	%
Shandong (rural areas)	210	142	67. 62	68	32. 38
Shandong (urban areas)	206	143	69. 42	63	30. 58
Zhejiang	150	97	64. 67	53	35. 33
Anhui	277	195	70. 40	82	29. 60
Ningxia	64	27	42. 19	37	57. 81

According to the literature review, almost all the provinces base their selections on experts' opinion in producing their respective lists of supplemented medicines, and a majority of experts are from the primary health-care facilities. At present, only a few provinces (e.g., Sichuan) apply the method of evidence-based medicine selection and consider the disease status in normal patients. (Tian, Song & Zhang, 2012) Under ideal conditions, the basis for the development of the EML should be evidence-based clinical practice guidelines. Currently, the existing clinical practice guidelines and medicines formularies are not widely and consistently used in practice. (Barber et al., 2013)

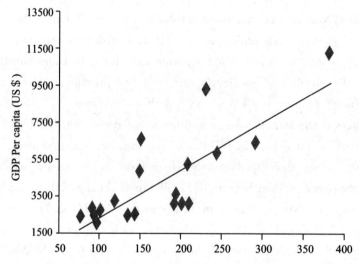

Figure 3-1　Correlation of GDP per capita and number of additional medicines (Wang & Zhang, 2011)

3.3　Centralized procurement

Before the reforms, procurement occurred at facility levels; primary health centers procured drugs directly from suppliers at variable prices. Following the implementation of NEMS, each province established unified bidding, purchasing and supply procedures for drugs sold in PHCs. A national guidance on centralized procurement of essential medicines at public health facilities was issued on November 19, 2010. By September 2011, government-led bidding platforms were established in all regions, and the majority of counties implemented online purchasing. The bidding announcement is usually published once a year. The manufacturers are the only tenders and have a responsible for the supply. In general, provincial procurement has promoted greater efficiencies in management. These efficiencies together with higher volume purchasing have resulted in reductions in medicines prices. The government reported that the tender price dropped on average by 33% compared to the last regional procurement; and declined by an average of 55% compared to national retail reference price. (China NDRC, 2011)

Anhui is the first to implement centralized procurement in China and provides a strong demonstration effect to other provinces. In Anhui, the purchasing center made a procurement plan according to the drug requirement from hospitals and issued public biding accordingly. During the tender process, a "two-envelope" tendering system is used, by which a tendering company would have to envelope and submit two sets of tendering documents: one for economic and technological specifications, and one for commercial transactions. The lowest price tenderer from those that qualify on technical assessment would be selected. Basically, for each medicine, no more than 3 forms are procured; and for each form, no more than 2 dosages procured. Anhui Model is being used by many provinces (including Shandong and Zhejiang). However, the specific measures in the procurement process are not uniform across the provinces. For instance, in Anhui, for the medicines with big demand, the provincial market is separated into several districts; and in each district one winner is selected for each medicine with specific form and dosage. However, in Shandong only one tender winner is selected for each medicine with specific form and dosage. So, the manufacturer would have 100% market share of the province if he wins. And in Zhejiang, for national essential medicines, one tender winner is selected for each medicine with specific form and dosage in whole provinces; and for provincial essential medicines, three winners are selected for each medicine with specific form and dosage. (Yang et al., 2012)

In addition, Shanghai Model is another representative, which focuses on medicine quality and patient demand. It constructs a comprehensive index system based on quality, price and market credit, with the ratio of 63%,

30%, and 7%, respectively. The selection is made according to the general score. Ningxia adopts this mode as well.

3. 4 Distribution and delivery

After the centralized bidding procurement, the selected manufacturers take responsibility to delivery medicines to health facilities directly. They are also allowed to entrust wholesale enterprises to distribute at the agreed bid prices. Currently, most provinces adopt the latter mode. Basically there are two arrangements for enterprises to participate in the delivery of medicines. One is the decentralized mode. The distribution market is open and all wholesale enterprises can participate in the delivery if they have a certain qualifications. Shandong is the representative of this mode. The other is the centralized mode. The distribution enterprises are selected through an open bidding process organized by the provincial government. The manufacturers make the choice within the list of winning enterprises. Zhejiang, Ningxia and Anhui all adopted this mode.

In general, provincial level distribution enterprises can deliver medicines throughout the province and municipal level distribution enterprises are only permitted to deliver within its distribution scope. The manufacturers can be entrusted to several wholesale enterprises, but each medicine is allowed to entrust only once. The provincial level distributors are encouraged to distribute directly. If not, they can make a sub-entrustment which however is allowed only once. Moreover, the primary distributors should take full responsibility for the sub-entrustment.

3. 5 Compensation for zero-profit policy

Regarding the compensation, China MoH issued a guideline about the reform of primary care facilities in February 2010 and indicated the compensation methods to recoup the revenue lost under the zero-profit policy. However, the announcement is less specific on how to operate. Therefore, arrangements for the compensation varies widely among regions. They can be generalized into four kinds (Wang et al., 2011; Yuan & Tang, 2012):

（1）The government makes separated management of revenues and expenditures. Beijing, Shanghai, and Jiangsu are the representatives. In this model, medicine sales revenues are returned to the county finance department. The institutions are then allocated budgets based on actual costs. It helps to cut off the interest link between hospital income, drug price and usage quantity. However, it also lows down hospital's enthusiasm for technical innovation.

（2）The compensation relies entirely on government subsidy. The allocation of government subsidies is based on prescription volumes and represents only the lost profit mark-up. Anhui, Ningxia and Shenzhen are the representatives. However, the perverse incentives (hospitals and doctors make money from selling medicines) are not removed in this case.

（3）Government substitutes subsidies with rewards based on the hospital's performance in the implementation of NEMS as well as the regional service population. Yunnan and Hunan are the representatives. However, it is difficult in practice for local authorities to get adequate data for the performance assessment.

（4）Multi-channel compensation. The compensation is mainly based on government subsidy and medical insurance fund, and supplemented by public health service subsidy, risk funds, medical services pricing adjustment, and so on. Shandong, Tianjin, Sichuan, and Liaoning are the representatives. This mode broadens the channels of compensation and makes good use of social resources. Recently, Anhui, Ningxia and Zhejiang have also begun to explore the multi-channel compensation.

In general, local governments are mainly responsible for replacing the revenues lost. (Barber et al., 2013) However, the subsidy level of local governments varies. Financially well-off eastern China enjoys better subsidies than comparatively poorer western areas.

3. 6　Summary

At present, the NEMS has been implemented in all provinces, providing practical benefits to local residents. In addition to 307 national essential medicines, 31 provinces establish provincial supplemented list according to their economic situation and specific health needs. The "two-envelope" tendering system is advocated by most provinces in the procurement process. Various distribution modes are used depending on local logistic capacity. The way of compensation for primary health care facilities needs to be further improved and the multi-channel compensation is currently the most popular mode.

Chapter 4　Impact on medicine prices and affordability

The rapid rise of medical and pharmaceutical expenditures has become a critical obstacle in accessing health care for the poor and its control is a key objective for health policy makers. (Maynard & Bloor, 2003) China is no exception. The high price of drugs has long been blamed for making medicine services unaffordable for less advantaged people and has triggered mounting complaints from the public. (Yu et al., 2010) This chapter is aimed to measure price changes of essential medicines in rural China before and after the implementation of NEMS and provide updated data on what people pay for medicines and how prices change with time, thereby evaluating the impact of NEMS on medicine access.

4. 1　Materials and methods

4. 1. 1　Drug inclusion criteria

Information of medicine prices was obtained from the four provinces studied through questionnaire survey (see Appendix II). In order to enable comparability, the medicines which fit the following conditions were under investigation. For each private facility in Zhejiang and Anhui, a medicine was selected, which was used both in Augusts of 2009 and 2010 and with the same strength and dosage form in these two periods. For each private facility in Shandong and Ningxia, a medicine was selected which was used in Junes of 2009, 2010 and 2011 and with the same strength and dosage form in these three periods.

Drugs (same chemical entity) with various strengths were dosage forms were considered as separate drugs in this study. All compared medicines were of the same generic name (might not come from the same producers). The quantity of drug usage was calculated in accordance with the pharmaceutical packaging units. For example, norfloxacin capsule is 0. 1g/tablet, packaging 12/board, and the amount of the drug is N board. The essential medicines include national essential medicines (NED) and provincial supplementary essential medicines (PED). Totally, 10,988 drugs were analyzed in this research, including 7,768 NEDs and 3,220 PEDs.

4.1.2 Individual price differences

Individual price differences were calculated for each drug before and after NEMS. The comparison was done through the percentage difference that may appear as a negative or positive value. Compared with the drug price in period 1, the percentage change of drug price in period 2 was calculated using Formula (1): $P \% = (P_2 - P_1)/P_1 \times 100\%$. Similarly, the percentage change of drug usage in period 2 was calculated using Formula (2): $Q \% = (Q_2 - Q_1)/Q_1 \times 100\%$.

The magnitude of the overall price change was calculated for three different lists: 2009-2010, 2010-2011, and 2009-2011. Due to the fact that individual price and quantity differences were abnormally distributed, we discussed them with a median value in this research and the 95% confidence interval of the median value was also calculated. Non-parametric test was used to compare differences between the groups or between the time periods. Pearson correlation test was used to test the significant or non-significant variations in relationships between price change and quantity change.

4.1.3 Price index

A real market always includes the sale of a vast number of goods. Economic theory defines price index to reflect what is happening to the overall level of prices in a given period of time. Economics calls a price with a fixed basket of goods Laspeyres index and a price index with a changing basket Paasche index. (Mankiw, 2007) In the case of a relatively short time (e.g., 10 years), a fixed basket of goods would not change. But with the variation of consumer preferences and social production capacity, the commonly used basket of goods would be changed. So the application of Laspeyres index and Paasche index can indicate the interactive relationship between the retail price and usage quantity. The Laspeyres index (P^{La}) and Paasche index (P^{Pa}) are calculated with Formula (3):

$$P^{La} = \frac{\sum\limits_{i=1}^{n} P_{2i}Q_{1i}}{\sum\limits_{i=1}^{n} P_{1i}Q_{1i}} \times 100\%$$

$$P^{Pa} = \frac{\sum\limits_{i=1}^{n} P_{2i}Q_{2i}}{\sum\limits_{i=1}^{n} P_{1i}Q_{2i}} \times 100\%$$

P_{1i} and P_{2i} stand for prices of drug i in periods 1 and 2; Q_{1i} and Q_{2i} stand for utilization of drug i in periods 1 and 2.

In this research, all the drugs can be regarded as a fixed basket of goods; and the drugs annual ranking of the top 50 according to usage quantity were regarded as the commonly used basket of goods of the year.

4.1.4 International price comparison

WHO/HAI method for international price comparison was used in this study. Twenty key medicines were picked up from the 10988 sample medicines. They are included in both WHO Global Core List (or Western Pacific Regional Core List) (HAI, 2008) and China NEML.

The medicine prices obtained during the survey are expressed as median price ratios (MPRs), or the ratio of a medicine's median unit price across outlets to the median unit price in the Management Sciences for Health Price Indicator Guide. The investigation was standardized at the year of 2009, using MSH 2009 international reference prices (IRP). (MSH, 2009) The year of 2009 was chosen as the base year. Patient price data are corrected for inflation or deflation between the survey year and the base year using the consumer price index (CPI) and also adjusted for the purchasing power parity (PPP) of the national currency. Therefore, MPR = [price / (1 + CPI)] * PPP / IRP. The CPI in 2010 is 3.3% (National Bureau of Statistics of China, 2010). The World Bank estimated that one US dollar was equivalent to about 4.42

Chinese yuan by PPP. (World Bank, 2010b) Generally, an MPR of 1 or less indicates an efficient public sector procurement system.

4.1.5 Medicine affordability

According to the WHO/HAI methodology, affordability was estimated by the number of days' incomes needed to purchase courses of treatment at common conditions. Treatment costs refer to medicines only and exclude the additional costs of consultation and diagnostic tests. In this study, the average daily income was considered using national relative poverty line which is 1,196 *yuan*/year (3.3 *yuan*/day) and per capita net income of rural households which is 5153 *yuan*/year (14.3 *yuan*/day). They respectively represent the low income population (LIP) and the middle income population (MIP). The figures are retrieved from the Ministry of Human Resources and Social Security. (MOHRSS, 2009) Treatments costing one day's income or less (for a 7-day supply for an acute condition, or a 30-day supply of medicine for chronic diseases) are generally considered affordable. (Ye et al.)

4.2 Results

4.2.1 Changes of drug prices

4.2.1.1 Individual price differences

In the comparison between 2009 and 2010, out of 10,988 drugs in this study, the prices of 9,747 (88.71%) drugs declined by 3983% (95% CI 38.78%-40%) and 1,057 (9.62%) drugs increased by 27.5% (95% CI 25%-32.35%). Overall, a median decrease of 34.38% (95% CI 30.36%-39.13%) in price was witnessed in 2010 as compared to the prices before NEMS implementation. NEDs decreased in price by 35.32% and the price of PEDs declined by 32.94%. The decrease in drug prices for NEDs was significantly higher than that for PEDs ($p < 0.05$). Moreover, the price of western medicines reduced by 41.62%, significantly higher than the decrease of TCMs ($p = 0.000$). Of each province studied, a significant difference ($p < 0.05$) is respectively observed between the 2009 prices and 2010 prices. Among them, the magnitude of price change in Shandong was the largest where the prices decreased by 40%. The highest price decrease after Shandong was seen in Anhui and Zhejiang. Ningxia was at the end of the scale and the prices fell by 4.76%. Results have been presented in Table 4-1 with price differences for all drugs and for drugs in various subcategories.

Table 4-1   Price differences for all drugs and for drugs
in various subcategories (2009-2010)

Category		N	Price (Yuan)		Price change		Quantity change	
			2009	2010	Median (%)	p	Median (%)	p
Category 1	WM	7,897	4.50	2.10	−41.62	0.000	0	0.000
	TCM	3,091	10.80	8.10	−24.32		12.50	
Category 2	NED	7,768	5.00	2.55	−35.32	0.027	0	0.136
	PED	3,220	9.00	5.50	−32.94		5.49	
Region	Shandong	7,897	3.50	1.85	−40.00	0.000	38.89	0.000
	Zhejiang	3,091	7.40	4.10	−33.62		5.5	
	Anhui	7,768	5.00	2.20	−37.00		0	
	Ningxia	3,220	2.63	2.40	−4.76		0	
Total		10,988	5.70	2.95	−34.38		1.52	

Note: p value, non-parametric test to test statistical difference of price change/quantity change within subcategories

Furthermore, Table 4-2 depicts the price changes of western medicines categorized according to the pharmacological classification listed in NEML. Among them, five categories are worthy of consideration (underscored in Table 4-2) because antimicrobial has the largest share of China drug market and occupies the largest proportion in China NEML; the cardiovascular, respiratory and digestive diseases have been the major disease burdens in China; and the nervous system diseases show an overall increase over the years. From Table 4-2, it is clear that the price decreases of these five categories are higher than the average level (34.38%) except the cardiovascular medicines. Table 4-3 depicts the price changes of TCMs categorized according to the functional classification listed in NEML.

Table 4-2　　Price changes of western medicines categorized according to
pharmacological classification（2009-2010）

Pharmacological classification	N	Price change (%)	Quantity change (%)
Antiallergics	121	−60.25	12.34
Blood-related medicine	317	−52.63	−5.00
Others	151	−50.00	0.00
Water-electrolyte-acid-base-balance medicine	842	−49.24	0.00
Antiparasitics	218	−48.90	6.79
Urinary system medicine	152	−48.76	6.26
Antimicrobial medicine	1,643	−46.88	0.00
Gynecological medicine	94	−46.72	2.08
Vitamin & mineral supplements	519	−43.57	−4.55
Antipsychotics	70	−42.30	−4.20
Ophthalmic medicine	177	−40.00	15.38
Dermatologic medicine	291	−39.53	0.00
Nervous system medicine	298	−39.07	0.00
Digestive system medicine	842	−38.89	2.04
Respiratory system medicine	333	−37.50	0.00
Hormone	489	−34.75	0.00
ENT medicine	38	−29.63	0.00
Antipyretic-analgesic and anti-inflammatory medicine	426	−29.41	1.61
Cardiovascular system medicine	805	−28.25	15.38
Biological medicine	72	72.22	−9.72

Table 4-3　　Price changes of TCMs categorized according to the
functional classification（2009-2010）

Pharmacological classification	N	Price change (%)	Quantity change (%)
Ophthalmic medicine	62	−35.44	7.27

Continued

Pharmacological classification	N	Price change (%)	Quantity change (%)
Internal medicine	2,309	−25. 58	12. 50
Surgical medicine	199	−25. 46	22. 22
Gynecological medicine	159	−24. 24	0. 00
Orthopedic medicine	288	−11. 59	10. 68
ENT medicine	74	−7. 44	9. 34

4. 2. 1. 2　Price elasticity of usage quantity

Compared with 2009, the overall quantity of drug usage increased by 1. 52% (95% CI 0. 00%-12. 5%) in 2010. However, considerable variation can be observed in the four provinces studied. The quantity of change in Shandong was the largest where the drug usage increased by 38. 89%. The next was Zhejiang (5. 5%). The median magnitude of quantity change in Anhui and Ningxia were both 0. Moreover, there was no significant difference between NED and PED in quantity change (p=0. 136). However, the increase in usage quantity for TCMs was significantly higher than that for Western medicines ($p = 0. 000$). In addition, among the five categories mentioned above, an extraordinary quantity difference was observed for cardiovascular system and digestive system medicines, increasing by 15. 38% and 2. 04% respectively.

In relation to price change, the drugs (N=4855) which decreased in price by 40% or increased in quantity by 5. 26%; the drugs (N = 2945) which decreased in price by 20%-40% grew in quantity by 4. 80%; and for drugs (N=3,188) which decreased in price by less than 20%, their median magnitude of quantity change was 0. Although the quantity change was not obvious in each subcategory, it still demonstrated a larger price decrease and quantity increase (χ^2 =96. 079, p=0. 000).

Regarding the relationship between price level and quantity change following the implementation of NEMS, the drugs retailing at more than 20 *yuan* (N=975) increased by 20. 51% in quantity; the drugs retailing at 10-20 *yuan* (N=1404) increased by 15. 57% in quantity; the drugs retailing at 2-10 *yuan* (N = 4420) showed an increase of 0. 06% in quantity; and the drugs retailing under 2 *yuan* (N=4189) showed no increase in quantity (see Table 4-4). So, it was clear that the higher the retail price, the larger the quantity increase ($\chi^2 = 75.930$, $p = 0.000$). In addition, Table 4-4 still reveals the price decrease was relatively low for high-priced drugs. For example, for drugs retailing under 2 *yuan*, their price decreased by 51.78%; however drugs retailing more than 20 *yuan* decreased in price by 16.33%.

Given such a price-elasticity, 100 out of 140 PHCs studied decreased drug sales by an average of 39% in 2010 compared with pre-NEMS. And among these 100 PHCs, 23 showed a decrease of less than 20% in drug sales; 29 decreased by 20%-40%; and 48 declined by 40% or above.

Table 4-4   Quantity changes for drugs retailing at different prices (2009-2010)

Pharmacological classification	N	Price change (%)	Quantity change (%)	
0-	4,189	−51.78	0.00	0.000
2-	4,420	−32.43	0.06	
10-	1,404	−23.63	15.57	
20-	975	−16.33	20.51	

Note: *p* value refers to statistical significance of relationship of price and quantity change

4.2.1.3 Further investigation in Shandong and Ningxia

To further explore the impact of NEMS on drug prices, the price differences in 2011 in Shandong and Ningxia were investigated. An overall decrease of 40% (95% CI 34.29%-43.74%) was observed between pre-NEMS (2009) prices and the prices in 2011. Figure 4-1 clearly demonstrates that the drug price declined annually from 2009 to 2011 ($p = 0.000$). In most cases, the drugs showed a very large decrease in 2010 and a modest decrease in 2011. Also, the prices of TCMs and WMs showed a similar decreasing trend ($p = 0.000$). The quantity of drug usage was increased by 32.20% in 2010 compared with 2009, and then increased by 6.58% in 2011. However, drug sales showed a continuous decrease from 2009 to 2011 with statistical significance ($p < 0.05$).

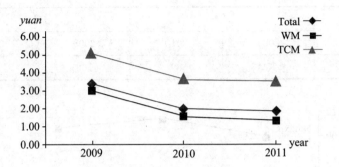

Figure 4-1   The evolution of drug prices in Shandong and Ningxia (2009-2011)

4. 2. 2   Analysis based on price index

Table 4-5 reveals the Laspeyres Index (P^{La}) and Paasche Index (P^{Pa}) of essential medicines in the four provinces studied. The value of P^{La} indicates that drug prices were lower than these before NEMS implementation, especially in Shandong, Zhejiang and Anhui. The P^{La} in Shandong declined to 62 in 2010 from 100 in 2009, indicating that drug prices decreased by 38%. The P^{La} in Zhejiang dropped to 64 in 2010, indicating that drug prices decreases by 36%. And the P^{La} in Anhui dropped to 52 in 2010, indicating that drug prices declined by 48%. However, the result of P^{Pa}, which indicates the price changes of the commonly used drugs, is not so optimistic. Its value was larger than P^{La} in each studied province. The P^{Pa} in Shandong was 75 in 2010 compared with 100 in 2009 and the prices only declined by 25%. The P^{Pa} in Zhejiang and Ningxia reached as high as 116 in 2010, suggesting an uptrend in prices. In addition, during 2009-2011 the P^{La} was always smaller than P^{Pa} from the observation in Shandong and Ningxia (see Figure 4-2).

Table 4-5   **Laspeyres Index and Paasche Index in the four**
provinces studied（2009-2010）

Region	P^{La}		P^{Pa}	
	2009	2010	2009	2010
Shandong	100	62	100	75
Zhejiang	100	64	100	116
Anhui	100	52	100	56

Continued

Region	P^{La}		P^{Pa}	
	2009	2010	2009	2010
Ningxia	100	89	100	116

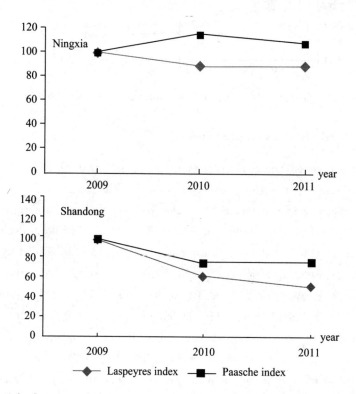

Figure 4-2   Laspeyres Index and Paasche Index in Shandong and Ningxia (2009-2011)

4. 2. 3   International price comparison

Before NEMS implementation, the MPR for the twenty observed essential medicines was 13. 858 times than the IRPs on average (see Table 4-6), Among them, the MPRs of six medicines were more than 10 times than their IRPs, with 69. 774 for diclofenac being the highest. Only two medicines, captopril (0. 600) and Nifedipine (0. 444), were at lower prices than the IRPs.

Table 4-6   Median price ratios for essential medicines before and after NEMS

Generic name	Strength	IRP (yuan)	No.of facilities	Before NEMS			After NEMS		
				Median price (yuan)	MPR	No.	Median price (yuan)	MPR	No.
Albendazole	200 mg	0.090	23	1.250	13.842	2,196	0.910	9.755	2,943
Amoxicillin	250 mg	0.087	62	0.289	3.322	710,965	0.148	1.647	1,023,859
Omeprazole	20 mg	0.044	62	0.443	9.995	192,025	0.462	10.089	122,101
Valproic acid	200 mg	0.061	4	0.130	2.131	3,048	0.113	1.800	3,200
Ibuprofen	600 mg	0.043	10	1.950	45.302	6,241	1.336	30.046	10,589
Ibuprofen	200 mg	0.038	33	0.060	1.579	228,935	0.030	0.764	265,522
Diazepam	5 mg	0.017	19	0.112	6.635	184,593	0.043	2.466	164,908
Metformin	500 mg	0.037	65	0.108	2.951	232,887	0.058	1.538	255,078
Ciprofloxacin	250 mg	0.101	33	0.325	3.222	55,588	0.100	0.960	232,518
Metronidazole	200-250 mg	0.025	66	0.050	1.975	195,917	0.031	1.183	276,410
Captopril	25 mg	0.067	63	0.040	0.600	734,983	0.026	0.370	943,724
Ranitidine	150 mg	0.088	57	0.133	1.508	147,694	0.059	0.651	140,302
Hydrochloro thiazide	25 mg	0.012	39	0.034	2.877	164,160	0.011	0.860	199,241
Diclofenac Sodium	50 mg	0.019	24	1.325	69.774	35,672	0.775	39.507	37,364
Cephalexin	250 mg	0.225	41	0.280	1.247	199,572	0.154	0.664	260,839
Ceftriaxone	1g/vial	1.802	65	10.000	5.550	80,783	1.731	0.930	95,416
Nifedipine	10 mg	0.074	38	0.033	0.444	591,005	0.012	0.156	608,764
Simvastatin	20 mg	0.121	39	4.657	38.586	26,256	2.486	19.940	48,700
Enalapril	10 mg	0.036	18	1.714	47.775	14,221	0.969	26.144	23,994
Enalapril	5 mg	0.045	13	0.798	17.841	93,310	0.675	14.608	82,796
Average					13.858			8.204	

Following the implementation of NEMS, the MPRs of all included medicines were declined except Omeprazole (ΔMPR = 0.094). Notably, the MPRs of four medicines were decreased by more than 10, including diclofenac, simvastatin, enalapril and ibuprofen (600mg). They were the most expensive medicines, ranking of the top 4 in 2009. On average, the MPR of the twenty medicines was 8.204 times than their corresponding IRPs after NEMS. Eight medicines were at lower prices than the IRPs; totally the prices of twelve medicines (about 60%) were less than two times higher than the reference price. However, still the prices of six medicines were more than 10 times higher than their IRPs, including omeprazole (10.089), ibuprofen (30.046), diclofenac (39.507), simvastatin (19.940), enalapril 10 mg (26.144) and enalapril 5 mg (14.608).

4.2.4 Medicine affordability

The affordability of medicines for rural residents before and after NEMS is listed in Table 1-4-7. On average, the medicines of standard treatment cost 1.76 days' incomes of MIP and 7.57 days' incomes of LIP in 2009. By 2010, the affordability of most medicines had been reasonable (with standard treatment costing a day's income or less) for MIP, except for ibuprofen (1.31 days' incomes), diclofenac (3.25 days' incomes), simvastatin (5.21 days' incomes) and enalapril (2.03-2.83 days' incomes). However, only nine medicines cost below a day's income of LIP. In general, the medicines cost 1.76 days' incomes of MIP and 4.21 days' incomes of LIP in 2010. Diclofenac, simvastatin and enalapril were the most costly for both MIP and LIP.

Table 4-7   Medicine affordability for rural residents before and after NEMS

Generic name	Strength	Median price (*yuan*)		DDD	Day	Days' income for MIP		Days' income for LIP	
		Before	After			Before	After	Before	After
Albendazole	200 mg	1.250	0.910	2	7	1.22	0.89	5.27	3.83
Amoxicillin	250 mg	0.289	0.148	3	7	0.42	0.22	1.83	0.94
Omeprazole	20 mg	0.443	0.462	1	30	0.93	0.97	4.00	4.17
Valproic acid	200 mg	0.130	0.113	3	30	0.82	0.71	3.52	3.06

Continued

Generic name	Strength	Median price (*yuan*)		DDD	Day	Days' income for MIP		Days' income for LIP	
		Before	After			Before	After	Before	After
Ibuprofen	600 mg	1. 950	1. 336	2	7	1. 91	1. 31	8. 22	5. 63

Generic name	Strength	Median price (*yuan*)		DDD	Day	Days' income for MIP		Days' income for LIP	
		Before	After			Before	After	Before	After
Ibuprofen	200 mg	0. 060	0. 030	4	7	0. 12	0. 06	0. 51	0. 25
Diazepam	5 mg	0. 112	0. 043	1	30	0. 23	0. 09	1. 01	0. 39
Metformin	500 mg	0. 108	0. 058	2	30	0. 45	0. 24	1. 95	1. 05
Ciprofloxacin	250 mg	0. 325	0. 100	2	7	0. 32	0. 10	1. 37	0. 42
Metronidazole	200-250 mg	0. 050	0. 031	6	7	0. 15	0. 09	0. 63	0. 39
Captopril	25 mg	0. 040	0. 026	2	30	0. 17	0. 11	0. 72	0. 47
Ranitidine	150 mg	0. 133	0. 059	2	30	0. 56	0. 25	2. 40	1. 07
Hydrochlor othiazide	25 mg	0. 034	0. 011	1	30	0. 07	0. 02	0. 31	0. 10
Diclofenac Sodium	50 mg	1. 325	0. 775	2	30	5. 55	3. 25	23. 93	14. 00
Cephalexin	250 mg	0. 280	0. 154	3	7	0. 41	0. 23	1. 77	0. 97
Ceftriaxone	1 g/vial	10. 000	1. 731	1	7	4. 89	0. 85	21. 07	3. 65
Nifedipine	10 mg	0. 033	0. 012	3	30	0. 21	0. 08	0. 89	0. 33
Simvastatin	20 mg	4. 657	2. 486	1	30	9. 76	5. 21	42. 05	22. 45
Enalapril	10 mg	1. 714	0. 969	1	30	3. 59	2. 03	15. 48	8. 75
Enalapril	5 mg	0. 798	0. 675	2	30	3. 35	2. 83	14. 41	12. 19
Average						1. 76	0. 98	7. 57	4. 21

4. 3　Discussion

4. 3. 1　NEMS and changes of medicine prices

One of the most important objectives of NEMS is to bring down the medicine prices. Results of this study indicates that the prices of 88. 71% of drugs decreased in 2010 and drug prices were 34. 38% lower than these before implementation of NEMS. This is in accordance with the NDRC report: "the drug prices in public primary health-care facilities decreased by about 30% in 2010" (Xinhuanet, 2010). The further investigation in Shandong and Ningxia also shows an overall decrease of 40% between 2009 prices and the prices in 2011. Therefore, NEMS had a positive effect on drug price control. Particularly, the largest price declines happened for anti-inflammatory and cardiovascular drugs. Considerable variation in price change was observed in the four provinces studied, reflecting differences in regulatory, economic and administrative contexts.

However, the MPR of medicine prices was still 8. 204 times higher than these of corresponding IRP in 2010. Given that an MPR of 1 or less indicates an efficient public sector procurement system, the medicine prices still have potential to drop. Take diclofenac, simvastatin, enalapril and ibuprofen for instance, their prices were more than 10 times lower than their IRPs in 2010. But it does not mean the lower the better. The excessive pursuit of lower prices might increase the following risks: Drugs may disappear in the market—the price is too low to discourage manufacturers and distributors to supply; Potential quality risks—the manufacturers may adulterate the quality to ensure the profit. (Song & Bian, 2012a).

4. 3. 2　Less expensive, but harder to find

The price index analysis shows the price changes in a different way. The value of P^{La} indicats the prices of the overall "basket" of medicines studied were much lower than these before NEMS implementation, especially in Shandong, Zhejiang and Anhui. However, the result of P^{Pa}, which indicates the price changes of the commonly used drugs, is not so optimistic. Its value is larger than P^{La} in each studied province and even reaches as high as 116 in Zhejiang and Ningxia. The situation is similar during 2009-2011 in Shandong and Ningxia. It suggests the commonly used drugs were always with higher prices or mild price reduction. Also, the results on the price elasticity of usage quality reveals the higher retail price and the larger quantity. Similar results are found in another survey in Shandong. (Yang et al.,2012)

The assumption of the policy design is that drug consumers would prefer drugs at a lower price. However, this does not take into account that drug prescriptions are written by doctors, not by the patients who will pay. The underlying motivations of doctors to use more expensive drugs may include: (1) The allocation of government subsidies in many regions (i.e. Anhui, Ningxia) was based on prescription volumes and represened only the lost profit mark-up. In this case, the perverse incentives for generating revenues from medicines were the same as these before the reform. (2) The financial incentives given by the manufacturers to the hospitals and doctors might have influenced the prescribing behaviors. (3) The profit margin of expensive drugs was relatively higher, which might encourage distributors to guarantee their supply. Due to the stock out or unresponsive supply of low-price drugs, doctors had to prescribe the expensive drugs. (Song & Bian, 2013a)

4.3.3 Increase in quantity, but low price elasticity

The results shows that the overall quantity of drug usage increased by 1.52% in 2010 compared with 2009. Also, the findings of the study demonstrate a larger price decrease and quantity increase. However, the price-elasticity of drugs was minor, which has been identified in prior studies (H. Zhu, 2004), so that the growth of drug quantity was not sufficient to make up the decline in medicine prices. Also, our finding shows the drug sales decreased 39% on average for the 149 PHCs studied in 2010. Given that medicine sales were the basis for operating costs for health facilities, the PHCs would suffer a substantial financial loss. Therefore, a closed eye must be kept on the compensation policy for primary health settings. The insufficient compensation may result in the shortage in routine operational activities, weak ability to maintain the essential medicine system, or sales of diagnostics, technologies, or other revenue generation methods to cover the basic operational costs.

4.3.4　Medicines unaffordable for low income population

The analysis on affordability shows the prices in relation to an individual's ability. The improved affordability found in the study supports the result that medicine prices were decreasing following the implementation of NEMS. In 2010, the medicines had reasonable affordability for MIP with standard treatment costing their 0.98 day's incomes. However, these medicines were still out-of-reach for LIP with standard treatment costing their 4.21 days' incomes on average. Meanwhile, even where individual treatments appear affordable, individuals or families who need multiple medications may quickly face unaffordable drug costs. An example is provided where the father has an ulcer and the child has infection and they are treated with omeprazole and ceftriaxone, respectively. If the family income is equivalent to the middle income population, medicine costs are 1.82 days' incomes. Therefore, social medical insurance should play an active role in ensuring affordability as well as access to medicines in addition to the further price control.

4.4　Summary

The introduction of NEMS was found to have a positive impact on containment of drug prices in rural primary health centers. Particularly, the largest price declines happened for anti-inflammatory and cardiovascular drugs. However, the current medicine prices remain higher compared to international reference prices. Medicines are often unaffordable for poor residents. The new shortage of some drugs occur. Sustainable mechanisms to compensate health-care providers for lost income are needed to ensure that NEMS is a success. Insurance expansion and comprehensive monitoring systems should be put into place to ensure equitable access to basic medical treatments, especially for the poor.

Chapter 5 Effect on improving rational drug use

All countries in the world, either rich or poor, have encountered problems with the insufficient use of good cost-effective drugs and the overuse of unnecessary drugs. (Pei, 2011) The medically inappropriate and economically inefficient use of drugs also occurs frequently in China. This chapter aims to examine the outcome of the NEMS objectives in terms of rational drug use in primary health-care facilities of China. Indicators of RDU were compared before and after policy implementation, and then discussed in regard to WHO standard or data from other research. The findings will provide quantitative baseline data for monitoring and improving prescribing processes in grass root level hospitals.

5.1 Materials and methods

5.1.1 Data sources

The materials were original outpatient prescriptions and prescription data were from primary care facilities in the four provinces studied. In Zhejiang and Anhui, the prescriptions were 100 randomly selected in 2009 and 2010 from each primary care facilities. In Shandong and Ningxia, the prescriptions were collected using systematic random sampling (at least ten prescriptions per month from January to June) in 2009, 2010 and 2011 from each facility. Data collection was anonymous (name or identifying information of the patients, general practitioners, and pharmacists were not obtained). The final data available for analysis consisted of 28,651 prescriptions, as shown in Table 5 1.

Table 5-1   The number of prescriptions collected from 146 PHCs in four provinces

	PHCs	Prescriptions		
		2009	2010	2011
Anhui	26	2,575	2,570	0
Zhejiang	87	8,408	8,700	0
Shandong	17	1,046	1,009	982
Ningxia	16	1,033	1,219	1,109
Total	146	13,062	13,498	2,091

5.1.2   Outcome measure

We extracted the data—the number of medicines, essential medicines and antibiotics, whether injections or hormones used and the total medical cost—from every individual prescription. The pretested indicators were described as below:

(1) Average number of drugs prescribed per encounter (ANDPE)

(2) Percentage of drugs prescribed from NEML (PEM)

(3) Average number of antibiotics prescribed per encounter (ANAPE)

(4) Percentage of encounters with an antibiotic prescribed (PEA)

(5) Percentage of encounters with an injection prescribed (PEI)

(6) Percentage of encounters with hormone prescribed (PEH)

5.1.3   Data analysis

Descriptive analyses of variables were carried out on the basis of means and corresponding percentages. The t-test was performed to compare the means and Fischer's exact test was to compare percentage distributions between two periods. The total medical cost per patient visit (TMC) was transformed into natural logarithms of the observation value to address the positive skew of the expenditure data. The relevant drug use indicators were computed as follows:

$$\text{ANDPE} = \frac{\text{total number of drugs prescribed}}{\text{total number of encounters surveyed}}$$

$$\text{PEM} = \frac{\text{total number of essential medicines prescribed} \times 100\%}{\text{total number of drugs prescribed}}$$

$$\text{ANAPE} = \frac{\text{total number of antibiotics prescribed}}{\text{total number of encounters surveyed}}$$

$$\text{PEA} = \frac{\text{number of patient encounters with an antibiotic} \times 100\%}{\text{total number of encounters surveyed}}$$

$$\text{PEI} = \frac{\text{number of patient encounters with an injection} \times 100\%}{\text{total number of encounters surveyed}}$$

$$\text{PEH} = \frac{\text{number of patient encounters with hormone} \times 100\%}{\text{total number of encounters surveyed}}$$

5. 2 Results

Table 5-2 shows the variables and changes in the use of essential medicines, antibiotics, injections and hormones for outpatient visits in 146 facilities from four surveyed provinces between 2009 and 2010.

Table 5-2   RDU indicators in 146 PHCs of the four surveyed provinces (2009-2010)

	Anhui			Zhejiang			Shandong			Ningxia			Total			Ideal
	2009	2010		2009	2010		2009	2010		2009	2010		2009	2010		value
ANDPE	4.17	4.25	+	3.57	3.3	− *	3.37	3.28	−	3.23	3.12	−	3.64	3.46	− *	2
PEM, %	75.62	86.88	+ *	61.31	83.29	+ *	50.65	49.41	−	55.35	60.59	+	63.33	79.89	+ *	100
ANAPE	0.96	1	+	0.79	0.75	− *	0.73	0.71	− *	0.72	0.81	+ *	0.81	0.8	−	
PEA, %	67.81	70.35	+ *	59.92	55.52	− *	51.43	51.54	+	53.15	60.38	+ *	60.26	58.48	− *	30
PEI, %	51.11	50.43	−	43.74	40.35	− *	30.59	29.04	−	28.36	27.97	−	42.93	40.31	− *	20
PEH, %	22.68	22.10	−	11.91	9.22	− *	11.09	10.70	−	1.65	2.30	+	13.15	11.16	− *	

+ : 2010-2009 > 0; − : 2010-2009 < 0

* : $p < 0.05$, p value refers to t-test to compare means or exact test to compare proportion distributions between the two periods

5. 2. 1 Medicines prescribed per encounter

Overall, the mean number of drugs prescribed per prescription decreased from 3.64 to 3.46 between 2009 and 2010. Fewer drugs were prescribed per consultation following the implementation of NEMS ($p < 0.01$). It was clear in Table 5-3 that the prescriptions where four or more drugs were prescribed decreased compared with 2009 ($p < 0.05$). In 2010, 15.1% of outpatient encounters were for one drug, 23.02% for two drugs, 20.98% for three drugs, and 40.91% for four or more. Moreover, on average 79.89% of drugs prescribed were from NEML in 2010 and in 2009 this proportion was 63.33%. The PEM in Zhejiang increased by 21.98%, more than any other province. Shandong was at the bottom end of the scale and only 49.41% of medicines were prescribed from NEML per encounter in 2010.

Table 5-3　Prescriptions by number of drugs per encounter, by year

No. of drugs per encounter	Prescriptions, N (%)		RD (95% CI)
	2009	2010	
0	2 (0.02)	4 (0.03)	0.01 (−0.02, +0.05)
1	1,745 (13.36)	2,036 (15.06)	+1.70 (+0.87, +2.54)
2	2,653 (20.31)	3,111 (23.02)	+2.71 (+1.72, +3.70)
3	2,657 (20.34)	2,836 (20.98)	+0.64 (−0.33, +1.61)
4	2,028 (15.53)	1,847 (13.67)	−1.86 (−2.71, −1.01)
5	1,796 (13.75)	1,660 (12.28)	−1.47 (−2.28, −0.66)
≥6	2,181 (16.70)	2,022 (14.96)	−1.74 (−2.62, −0.86)

Note: RD means the difference of proportion between the years; CI means confidence interval

5.2.2　Antibiotics use

In this survey, 60.26% of all outpatient encounters were prescribed one or more antibiotic in 2009, which decreased to 58.48% in 2010 ($p < 0.01$). However, it should be noted that the rates were increasing in Anhui, Shandong and Ningxia. Overall, the mean number of antibiotics prescribed per encounter was 0.8 in 2010, almost equal to 0.81 in 2009. The antibiotics prescribed per encounter were reduced in Zhejiang and Shandong. The absence of a clear benefit was because more antibiotics per encounter were prescribed in Anhui and Ningxia. In addition, it was clear in Table 5-4 that 2.08% of all prescriptions contained three or more kinds of antibiotics in 2009; this proportion increased to 2.26% in 2010 ($p < 0.05$).

Table 5-4   Prescriptions by number of antibiotics per encounter (2009-2010)

No. of drugs per encounter	Prescriptions, N (%)		RD (95% CI)
	2009	2010	
No antibiotics	5,191(39.74)	5,612(41.52)	+1.78 (+0.60, +2.96)
With antibiotics	7,871(60.26)	7,904(58.48)	−1.78 (−2.96, −0.60)
1	5,450(41.72)	5,403(39.97)	−1.75 (−3.28, −0.22)
2	2,149(16.45)	2,195(16.24)	−0.21 (−1.36, +0.94)
⩾3	272(2.08)	306(2.26)	+0.18 (−0.27, +0.63)

Note: RD means the difference of proportion between the years; CI means confidence interval

5.2.3   Injection and hormone use

The rates of prescriptions containing injections reduced in all selected provinces between 2009 and 2010. On average 40.31% of consultations resulted in an injection in 2010, with 27.97% for Ningxia being the lowest. Also, hormone use improved significantly and the percentage of patients prescribed hormones declined to 11.16% in 2010.

5.2.4   Further investigation in Shandong and Ningxia

5.2.4.1   Drug prescribing indicators

The drug prescribing in 2011 was further investigated in Shandong and Ningxia. The results on drug use are showed in Table 5-5. It reveals that the rate of medicines prescribed from NEML increased annually since the implementation of NEMS ($p < 0.01$). Significantly fewer prescriptions where an antibiotic was prescribed were found in 2011 and the average number of antibiotics prescribed per encounter was also significantly lower ($p < 0.01$). Analysis of data also indicates that fewer outpatient encounters resulted in prescribed injections ($p < 0.01$). Injections (excluding TCM injections) prescribed mainly referred to: solutions correcting water, electrolyte and acid-base disturbance (35.20%), Antimicrobials (23.1%), vitamins and minerals (9.7%), Antiviral medicines (7.3%), hormones (5.1%). however, the ANDPE and PEH did not present a clear benefit in 2011compared to 2009 with the available data.

Table 5-5   RDU indicators in 33 PHCs of Shandong and Ningxia（2009-2011）

	Shandong			Ningxia			Total			Ideal value
	2009	2010	2011	2009	2010	2011	2009	2010	2011	
ANDPE	3.37	3.28	3.36	3.23	3.12	3.15	3.30	3.19	3.25	2
PEM，%	50.65	49.41	65.67	55.35	60.59	70.64	53.03	55.49	68.31	100
ANAPE	0.73	0.71	0.66	0.72	0.81	0.70	0.73	0.77	0.68	
PEA，%	51.43	51.54	47.15	53.15	60.38	54.19	52.28	56.37	50.88	30
PEI，%	30.59	29.04	26.68	28.36	27.97	22.36	29.50	28.50	24.40	20
PEH，%	11.09	10.70	11.20	1.65	2.30	1.89	6.40	6.10	6.30	

5.2.4.2 Total medical cost per patient visit

Cost analysis in Shandong and Ningxia reveals that theTMC significantly increased from 25.77 to 27.09 *yuan*（$p<0.01$）during 2009-2011, as shown in Figure 5-1. From Table 5-6, it is easy to see that the majority of prescriptions（$>50\%$）were cost below 20 *yuan*. However, the prescription where TMC was over 50 *yuan* remained common.

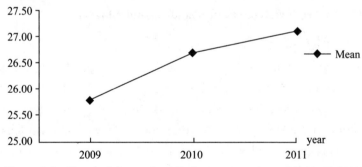

Figure 5-1   Trend of the total medical cost per patient visit（2009-2011）

Table 5-6   Medical cost per patient visit in ten *yuan* intervals（2009-2011）

Cost（*yuan*）	2009		2010		2011	
	Frequency	%	Frequency	%	Frequency	%
0-	592	28.5	599	26.9	479	22.9
10-	544	26.2	583	26.2	569	27.2
20-	364	17.5	402	18.0	403	19.3

Continued

Cost (*yuan*)	2009		2010		2011	
	Frequency	%	Frequency	%	Frequency	%
30-	213	10. 2	262	11. 8	257	12. 3
40-	137	6. 6	149	6. 7	135	6. 5
50-	88	4. 2	64	2. 9	84	4. 0
60-	55	2. 6	52	2. 3	51	2. 4
70-	25	1. 2	36	1. 6	32	1. 5
80-	14	0. 7	16	0. 7	20	1. 0
90-	13	0. 6	10	0. 4	13	0. 6
100-	34	1. 6	55	2. 5	48	2. 3
Total	2,079	100. 0	2,228	100. 0	2,091	100. 0

Furthermore, the cost of encounter where an injection was prescribed was significantly higher than that where no injection was prescribed ($p=0.000$). Similarly, the cost of encounter where antibiotics were prescribed was also significantly higher than that where no antibiotics was prescribed ($p=0.000$) (see Table 5-7).

Table 5-7   Medical cost per patient visit by different medicine use patterns

		Prescription cost (*yuan*)		Z	*p*
		Mean	Sd		
Injection use	Yes	36. 936	45. 899	−17. 458	0. 000
	No	22. 579	23. 825		
Antibiotics use	Yes	27. 127	28. 731	−7. 389	0. 000
	No	25. 847	35. 568		

Note: *p* value refers to Mann-Whitney test

In addition, the TMC was transformed into natural logarithms of the observation value and addressed a positive skew distribution where the mean was 2. 83 and 95% CI was 2. 81-2. 85, as shown in Figure 5-2. That is to say, the prescription costing 16. 53-17. 37 *yuan* (the corresponding observation value of 95% CI) or less was reasonable.

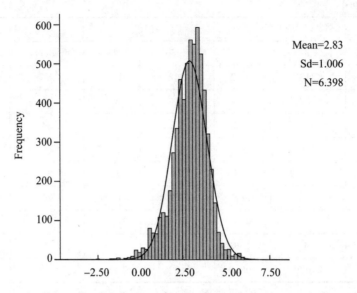

Figure 5-2　Frequency distribution of medical cost per patient visit (logarithms)

5. 3　Discussion

Prescribing practices among the surveyed regions appeared to have improved after the introduction of NEMS. Firstly, the study reveals that fewer drugs were prescribed per consultation ($p < 0.01$). In 2010, patients were prescribed on average 3. 46 drugs per prescription, which was however still double than the derived WHO standard value of 1. 6-1. 8 (Isah et al., 2006) and also higher than the average of 2. 2 found in a study of 17 developing countries where the highest recorded is 3. 8, (Pavin et al., 2003). Thus, the results indicate that the trend towards polypharmacy still exists in China and it is among the world's most severe cases. Such a trend might be attributed to the provider-induced consumption, because the allocation of government subsidies in many facilities was based on prescription volumes and the distorted incentives for generating hospital revenues from medicines were not eliminated. Another possible factor could be that patients influence the decision-making process. Patients believe that prescribing more drugs can ensure improvement and facilitate the cure of their conditions more quickly.

(Soumerai, 1998) Furthermore, "bargain mentality" also encourages the irrational use. In some regions (such as Ningxia), there is an annual medical compensation (about 30 *yuan* per person) for outpatient services. Patients prefer to get medicines for free and always ask physicians to prescribe medicines within the quota especially at the end of the fiscal year, no matter whether they are needed.

Secondly, analysis of the data reveals that essential medicines constituted a reasonably high proportion of the medicines prescribed in PHCs. On average 80% of drugs prescribed appeared on NEML in 2010. This result indicates essential medicines were being recognized and widely used. A recent study covering 18 medicines in 17 largely middle-income countries shows that costs to patients could be reduced by an average of 60% by switching from originator brands to the lowest priced generic equivalents (Cameron, 2010). So, the priority of essential medicines could help improve medicine access and is worth advocating. However, the exclusive use in PHCs should be considered. The existence of a reasonable complete list that suggests the best treatment therapy for every patient is impossible because of the limitation of categories and the number of essential medicines. (Tian et al., 2012) This practice can also cause conflicts between the prescription of doctors and the medical needs of patients.

Thirdly, the study shows that the number of outpatient encounters where one or more antibiotics were prescribed decreased to 58.48% in 2010 ($p<0.01$), whereas the number recommended by WHO is 20.0%-26.8% (WHO, 1993b). Moreover, we found no evidence to show any decline in the mean number of antibiotics prescribed per encounter. So, the findings regarding antibiotics use were not encouraging. Antibiotics are essential but their overuse can increase antibiotic resistance, which will endanger the therapeutic effectiveness, increase treatment failure and, as a result, lead to longer and more severe illness episodes with higher costs and mortality rate. (WHO, 2001b) The major factors that influence high percentage of antibiotics prescribed in China might be a lack of knowledge about appropriate antibiotic use, including overestimation of the severity of illness to justify antibiotic prescribing by physicians, and pressure from patients who believe that antibiotics provide rapid symptomatic relief of the disease. (Desalegn, 2013;

Quick，2003）

Fourthly，the results show that the injection and hormone use improved significantly. The percentage of prescriptions with injections in Shandong and Ningxia in 2011 was 24.4%, which was higher than that reported in 35 developing countries（22.8%）.（WHO，2004c）Moreover，it has been recommended that fewer than 20% of prescriptions should include injections.（Deepak，2006）In China，the mistaken belief that "Injections mean you will get well sooner" always makes patients request an injection. Relative to oral drug therapy，injections are more expensive because of the additional cost of syringes，sterilization control，and well-trained personnel. In addition to increase the economic burden of patients，overuse of injections also runs the risk of unsafe needles that can increase the transmission of AIDS，hepatitis B and C，and other blood-borne diseases.（Zhuo，Sleigh & Wang，2002）Notably in our survey，23.1% of injections were prescribed for antimicrobial，which could increase the risk of antibiotic resistance.

Finally，cost analysis in Shandong and Ningxia reveals that the TMC significantly increased during 2009-2011（$p < 0.01$）. After the introduction of NEMS，centralized procurement has promoted greater efficiency in management. This together with zero-profit drug policy has resulted in reductions in medicine prices. However medical costs did not drop correspondingly. The poor outcome might be partly due to the irrational use of medicines.（Song & Bian，2012b）Our findings indicate that the medical cost per encounter with antibiotics or injections was higher than that without，which is consist with other research（e. g. Xu，Fang & Jiang，2011）. Furthermore，this study derives the prescription costing 16.53-17.37 *yuan* or less was reasonable，which could provide a scientific reference for the cost control.

Promoting the rational use of drugs has never been an easy task. It requires interventions on both providers and consumers. Education can make a difference. One study shows that doctors with a bachelor level medical training are less likely to prescribe injections than those with only vocational level training.（Dong，Wang，Gao & Yan，2011）Another simulated patient study shows that patient knowledge regarding the appropriate use of antibiotics can effectively reduce both antibiotic prescriptions and drug expenditure for identical complaints. (Currie, 2010) In addition, where profits from selling drugs have been eliminated, appropriate financial compensation mechanisms are needed to ensure a sustainable development of the primary care facilities. (Yang et al., 2012)

5. 4 Summary

There is a positive association between NEMS and more appropriate use of medications in primary care settings in China. The declines were recorded in the mean number of drugs prescribed per patient and the proportion of patients being prescribed antibiotics. Increases in the utilization of essential medicines have occurred. Also, the injection and hormone use were improved significantly. However, the over-prescription of antibiotics and injections as well as polypharmacy were common. There is still a large unfinished agenda and policy improvement is needed.

Chapter 6   Impact on primary
health-care facilities

6. 1   Introduction

The NEMS tackles the problem of access to appropriate medicines for 1. 3 billion Chinese people by focusing on providing essential medicines to all. This policy has now been implemented in all government-run primary level facilities. Great efforts have been made to encourage utilization of essential medicines and services at primary levels. To trace the availability of essential medicines in these settings will help to improve the program's performance. In addition, drug sales revenues are to be replaced by the NEMS and the shift inevitably leads to a drop in income for hospitals. Therefore, how to make essential medicines benefit the public without the bankruptcy of grassroots health facilities is currently a critical issue.

This chapter is aimed to present evidences on impact of NEMS using hospitals as the basis of the analysis. It focuses on the availability of essential medicines and the financial operational activities of hospitals. Importantly, it explored the feasible measures of hospital compensation based on SD approach. Combining case study and SD approach as proposed by the Dynamic Synthesis Methodology (DSM) is beneficial in that the strength of the case study enables the collection of data in its natural setting.

6. 2　New characteristic of primary health-care facilities under NEMS

6. 2. 1　Method

6. 2. 1. 1　Data sources

Data was obtained from field survey in 36 PHCs in Shandong and Ningxia. A self-compiled questionnaire was used to collect information on hospital operational activities during 2008-2011 (see Appendix I). Key informant interview was performed to provide supplementary information for quantitative investigation.

6. 2. 1. 2　Data analysis

Descriptive analyses of variables were carried out on the basis of means and corresponding percentages. For group comparisons, a one-way ANOVA test was used whenever possible.

The availability of essential medicines refers to the number of essential medicines stocked at individual facilities divided by the total number of medicines in the EML. The response rate of medicine delivery (RR) is determined by dividing delivery frequency of distributors by the order frequency of PHCs. The arrival rate of medicines (AR) is determined by dividing the number of medicine actually arrived in PHCs by the number of medicines ordered by PHCs. All these three indicators are expressed in the form of percentage.

6. 2. 2　Results

6. 2. 2. 1　The availability of essential medicines

The amount of medicines stocked in the 36 PHCs decreased after the introduction of NEMS ($p=0.108$), as shown in Figure 6-1. The quantity in 2011 was about 343 on average, a 25.67% reduction compared with 2009. However, the percentage of essential medicines stocked at hospitals obviously increased and reached 100% after 2009. Table 6-1 lists the availability of essential medicines in PHCs during 2009-2011. The availability of NEDs increased annually ($p=0.381$). In 2011, the mean availability was 72.58±20.26% for NEDs and 61.09±19.36 for

PEDs. Overall the mean availability of essential medicines in PHCs had reached as high as 66.83% by 2011.

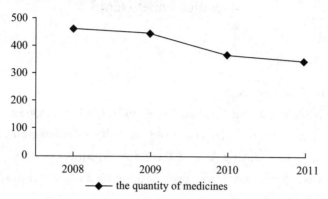

Figure 6-1   The quantity of medicines stocked in PHCs (2008-2011)

Table 6-1   **The availability of essential medicines in PHCs (2009-2011)**

	Availability of NEDs, %			Availability of PEDs, %			Total, %		
	Mean	Sd	95% CI	Mean	Sd	95% CI	Mean	Sd	95% CI
2009	61.95	24.2	44.64-79.27	75.35	38.21	45.98-104.72	68.30	31.45	53.14-84.46
2010	69.22	19.43	61.54-76.91	61.77	21.89	52.93-70.61	65.57	20.81	59.83-71.30
2011	72.58	20.26	64.56-80.59	61.09	19.36	53.43-68.75	66.83	20.46	61.25-72.42
p	0.38			0.27			0.89		

Note: p value refers to one-way ANOVA for trend

6.2.2.2   The efficiency of medicine delivery

Table 6-2 shows the evolution of the efficiency of medicine delivery during 2009-2011, which is embodied by RR and AR. A downward trend was observed in the two indicators after the implementation of NEMS, though there was no statistical significance ($p = 0.631$ for RR, 0.753 for AR). In 2011, the RR was 97.56±10.28% and the AR was 86.45±27.49%.

Table 6-2   **The efficiency of medicines delivery for PHCs (2009-2011)**

	Response rate of delivery, %			Arrival rate of medicines, %		
	Mean	Sd	95% CI	Mean	Sd	95% CI
2009	99.68	1.63	99.02-100.34	91.66	21.95	81.08-102.24

Continued

	Response rate of delivery, %			Arrival rate of medicines, %		
	Mean	Sd	95% CI	Mean	Sd	95% CI
2010	97. 67	11. 49	93. 38-101. 96	90. 33	21. 41	81. 29-99. 37
2011	97. 56	10. 28	93. 72-101. 39	86. 45	27. 49	74. 84-98. 06

6. 2. 2. 3　The uptake of health services

The number of patient visits in PHCs presented an upward trend at the post-implementation period (see Figure 6-2). Outpatient (including emergency) visits in 2011 was 47,353 with an increase of 11. 58% from 2009 (p for trend$=0. 995$ for 2008-2011); and inpatient admissions in 2011 was 2,518, an increase of 31. 10% from 2009 (p for trend$=0. 056$ for 2009-2011).

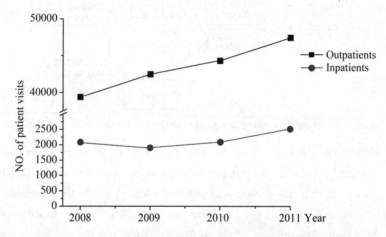

Figure 6-2　The number of patient visits in PHCs (2008-2011)

6. 2. 2. 4　Hospital income and expenditure

The components and their interrelation of hospital income and expenditure in primary health-care facilities are presented in Figure 6-3 (China MoF and MoH, 2010). Hospital incomes include government subsidy, medical service income, drug income and other income. Hospital expenditures include capital construction expense, medical service expense, drug expense and other expense. The net revenue of hospital is the balance of hospital income after deducting hospital expenditure.

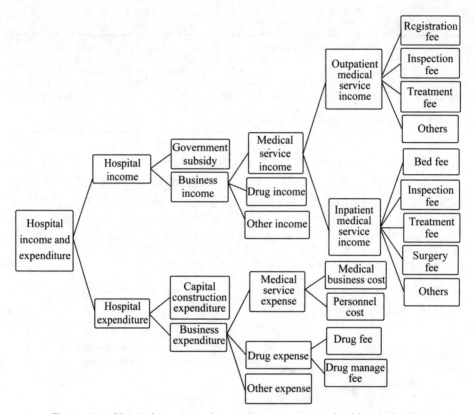

Figure 6-3　Hospital income and expenditure in primary health care facility

In this survey, the hospital income rose from 434. 15 thousand *yuan* in 2009 to 539. 48 thousand *yuan* in 2011, with an increase of 24. 26%. However, the hospital revenue reduced during this process and incurred a loss of 21. 79 thousand *yuan* (see Table 6-3). Figure 6-4 details the changing income structure of the health facility. It is clear that drug income as a proportion of total income declined after the implementation of the NEMS and dropped to 29. 65% in 2011. In the meanwhile, the percentage of total income supplied by the government increased and reached 28. 37% in 2011.

Table 6-3　　Income and expenditure of PHCs (2009-2011, thousand *yuan*)

Year	Income per hospital	Expenditure per hospital	Hospital net revenue
2009	434. 15	416. 36	17. 79
2010	509. 69	520. 64	−10. 95
2011	539. 48	561. 27	−21. 79

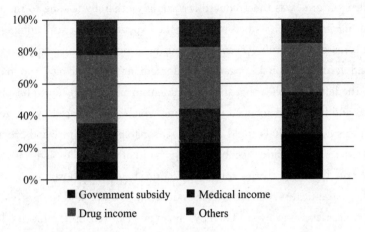

Figure 6-4　Changes of hospital income structure (2009-2011)

6.3　Tentative compensation for primary care facilities: a SD approach

A system dynamic model of hospital operation (HO model) was developed and simulated with Vensim software 5.1 to explore the feasible solutions for hospital compensation in the context of new health care reform.

6.3.1　A systematic dynamic model of hospital operation

6.3.1.1　Data sources

Information about hospital operation (HO) was collected from PHCs in Shandong and Ningxia and a mean value was used in the analysis. The data in 2010 was assigned as the initial value. Its rate of change from 2010 to 2011 was used to predict the future value. The values of some constant variables were obtained from national health statistics yearbook due to the poor availability in the on-site survey i.e. percentage of drug management fee. The healthcare reform is on-going and policies may change frequently. To ensure reliable and realistic, the simulation was set from 2011 to 2015 and the step was 0.5 year.

6.3.1.2　Causal loop diagram

The causal loop about hospital income and expenditure in the context of NEMS is illustrated in Figure 6-5. There are three feedback loops in this diagram. The first is a positive reinforcement (marked by "+") loop on the right. It indicates that the NEMS made efforts to cancel drug markups and then to reduce medicine prices and hospital drug income was then reduced accordingly, thereby leading to the reduction of hospital income; hospitals had to reduce the expenditure correspondingly in order to ensure a reasonable profit, eventually causing a decline in the quality of service. The second feedback loop is negative reinforcement ("balancing" and marked by "−") on the left. It implies that the government increased subsidy to hospitals after the reform and hospitals recouped the revenue which was replaced by the zero-profit policy; in this case hospitals could ensure a reasonable expenditure and provide high-quality services. The third feedback loop is in the middle and also negative reinforcement. It reflects a price compensation mechanism for hospitals. In this loop, a fixed pharmaceutical service fee was introduced to hospital and the price-setting for medical services was improved. Thereby, hospitals can recoup the income loss, and ensure the reasonable expenditures as well as health services of high quality.

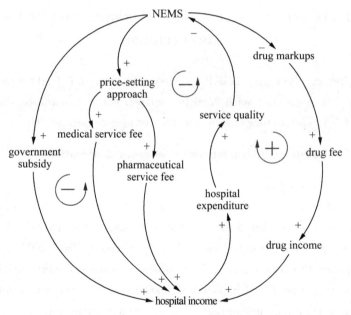

Figure 6-5   Causal loop diagram of hospital operation in the context of NEMS

6.3.1.3   Stock and flow diagram

A stock and flow diagram was then developed to perform a more detailed quantitative analysis based on the causal loop diagram. It contained four sectors in this study: drug income sector, medical service income sector, government subsidy sector and hospital expenditure sector, as shown in Figure 6-6. Table 6-4 lists the key variables and equations used in the stock and flow diagram.

(1)Drug income sector

Drug income includes outpatient and inpatient drug income. Under medicine zero-profit policy, it is equal to drug procurement cost. In hospital operation, drug income is determined by average drug fee per patient visit multiplying the number of patients. Notably, we assumed NEMS could reduce average drug fee per patient visit by 3% a year. This figure was based on a research in Japan which implies that the expenditures on drugs for patients are inflated by substitution into high-price, high-markup drugs by 4.4% and overuse of drugs by 10.6%. (Iizuka, 2007) It can thus be concluded that drug fee would drop by 15% if the providers' induced demand is completely eliminated. Since it could not be achieved overnight and China's situation might be more serious, we suppose the average drug fee per patient visit declined by 3% annually and the overall decline could reached about 15% in five years.

(2)Medical service income sector

Medical service income refers to outpatient and inpatient medical service income. It is determined by average medical service fee per patient visit multiplying the number of patients. Generally, the average medical service fee per outpatient includes registration fee, treatment fee, inspection fee and other fees (such as material fee). The average medical service fee per inpatient includes treatment fee, surgery fee, inspection fee, bed fee and other inpatient fees. All the fee units are supposed to grow exponentially.

(3)Government subsidy sector

Government subsidy is another important income source of hospitals. In Shandong and Ningxia, the government subsidy showed a 15% annual growth in the post-implementation period of NEMS.

(4)Hospital expenditure sector

Hospital expenditure includes medical expense, drug expense and capital construction expenditure. Medical expense refers to personnel expense and medical business expense. Drug expense includes drug procurement cost and drug management fee. Among them, procurement cost is equal to drug income. Drug management fee constitutes 17% of total drug expense according to China Health Statistical Yearbook. (Chinese MoH, 2011a)

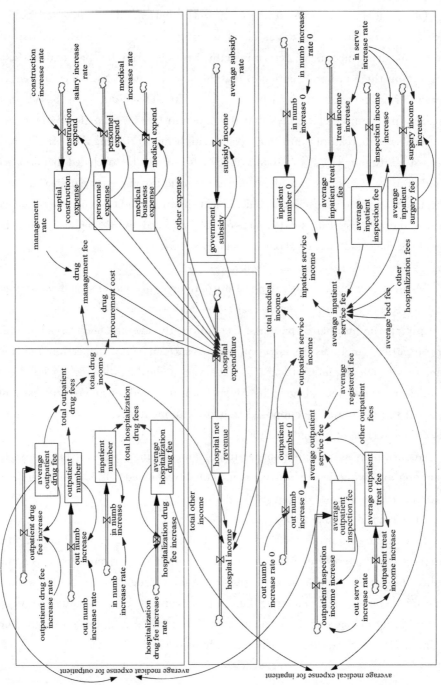

Figure 6-6 Stock and flow diagram of hospital operation under NEMS

Table 6-4   Key variables and equations in the stock and flow diagram

No.	Variable and SD equation (or value)	Unit	Variable type
1	final time＝2015	year	Initial
2	initial time＝2010	year	Initial
3	time step＝0. 5	year	Initial
4	initial outpatient number＝4. 4315	ten thousand people	Initial
5	initial inpatient number＝0. 2115	ten thousand people	Initial
6	initial average outpatient drug fee＝32. 56	*yuan* per capita	Initial
7	initial average hospitalization drug fee＝265. 11	*yuan* per capita	Initial
8	initial capital construction expense＝19. 24	ten thousand *yuan*	Initial
9	initial personnel expense＝154. 97	ten thousand *yuan*	Initial
10	initial medical business expense＝76. 9	ten thousand *yuan*	Initial
11	initial average outpatient inspection fee＝5. 1	*yuan* per capita	Initial
12	initial average outpatient treat fee＝5. 63	*yuan* per capita	Initial
13	initial average inpatient treat fee＝116. 15	*yuan* per capita	Initial
14	initial average inpatient inspection fee＝45. 28	*yuan* per capita	Initial
15	initial average inpatient surgery fee＝61. 28	*yuan* per capita	Initial
16	initial government subsidy＝118. 045	ten thousand *yuan*	Initial
17	initial hospital income＝14. 105	ten thousand *yuan*	Initial
18	out numb increase rate＝0. 069	dmnl	Constant
19	in numb increase rate＝0. 19	dmnl	Constant
20	outpatient drug fee increase rate＝－0. 03	dmnl	Constant
21	hospitalization drug fee increase rate＝－0. 03	dmnl	Constant
22	drug management rate＝0. 17	dmnl	Constant
23	construction increase rate＝0. 078	dmnl	Constant
24	salary increase rate＝0. 21	dmnl	Constant
25	medical increase rate＝0. 21	dmnl	Constant
26	out serve increase rate＝0. 0843	dmnl	Constant
27	average registered fee＝0. 3	*yuan* per capita	Constant

Continued

No	Variable and SD equation (or value)	Unit	Variable type
28	in serve increase rate=0.036	dmnl	Constant
29	average bed fee=45	*yuan* per capita	Constant
30	average subsidy rate=0.15	dmnl	Constant
31	outpatient number=INTEG(out numb increase, initial outpatient number)	ten thousand people	Level
32	inpatient number = INTEG (in numb increase, initial inpatient number)	ten thousand people	Level
33	average outpatient drug fee=INTEG (outpatient drug fee increase, initial average outpatient drug fee)	*yuan* per capita	Level
34	average hospitalization drug fee=INTEG (hospitalization drug fee increase, initial average hospitalization drug fee)	*yuan* per capita	Level
35	capital construction expense=INTEG (construction expend, initial capital construction expense)	ten thousand *yuan*	Level
36	personnel expense = INTEG (personnel expense, initial personnel expense)	ten thousand *yuan*	Level
37	medical business expense=INTEG (medical expense, initial medical business expense)	ten thousand *yuan*	Level
38	average outpatient inspection fee=INTEG (outpatient inspection income increase, initial average outpatient inspection fee)	*yuan* per capita	Level
39	average outpatient treat fee=INTEG (outpatient treat income increase, initial average outpatient treat fee)	*yuan* per capita	Level
40	average inpatient treat fee=INTEG (treat income increase, initial average inpatient treat fee)	*yuan* per capita	Level

Continued

No.	Variable and SD equation (or value)	Unit	Variable type
41	average inpatient inspection fee＝INTEG (inspection income increase, initial average inpatient inspection fee)	*yuan* per capita	Level
42	average inpatient surgery fee＝INTEG (surgery income increase, initial average inpatient surgery fee)	*yuan* per capita	Level
43	government subsidy＝INTEG (subsidy income, initial government subsidy)	ten thousand *yuan*	Level
44	hospital net revenue＝INTEG (hospital income－ hospital expenditure, initial hospital net revenue)	ten thousand *yuan*	Level
45	outpatient drug fee increase＝average outpatient drug fee * outpatient drug fee increase rate	*yuan*/year	Rate
46	out numb increase＝outpatient number * out numb increase rate	ten thousand people/year	Rate
47	in numb increase＝inpatient number * in numb increase rate	ten thousand people/year	Rate
48	hospitalization drug fee increase＝average hospitalization drug fee * hospitalization drug fee increase rate	*yuan*/year	Rate
49	construction expend＝capital construction expense * construction increase rate	ten thousand *yuan*/year	Rate
50	personnel expend ＝ personnel expense * salary increase rate	ten thousand *yuan*/year	Rate
51	medical expend ＝ medical business expense * medical increase rate	ten thousand *yuan*/year	Rate
52	outpatient inspection income increase ＝ average outpatient inspection fee * out serve increase rate	*yuan*/year	Rate
53	outpatient treat income increase ＝ average outpatient treat fee * out serve increase rate	*yuan*/year	Rate

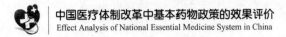
Continued

No.	Variable and SD equation (or value)	Unit	Variable type
54	treat income increase = average inpatient treat fee * in serve increase rate	*yuan*/year	Rate
55	inspection income increase = average inpatient inspection fee * in serve increase rate	*yuan*/year	Rate
56	surgery income increase = average inpatient surgery fee * in serve increase rate	*yuan*/year	Rate
57	subsidy income = government subsidy * average subsidy rate	ten thousand *yuan*/year	Rate
58	hospital income = government subsidy + total drug income + total medical income + total other income	ten thousand *yuan*/year	Rate
59	hospital expenditure = personnel expense + medical business expense + drug procurement cost + drug management fee + capital construction expense + other expense	ten thousand *yuan*/year	Rate
60	total outpatient drug fees = average outpatient drug fee * outpatient number	ten thousand *yuan*	Auxiliary
61	total hospitalization drug fees = average hospitalization drug fee * inpatient number	ten thousand *yuan*	Auxiliary
62	total drug income = total hospitalization drug fees + total outpatient drug fees	ten thousand *yuan*	Auxiliary
63	drug procurement cost = total drug income	ten thousand *yuan*	Auxiliary
64	drug management fee = total drug income * drug management rate	ten thousand *yuan*	Auxiliary
65	average outpatient service fee = average outpatient inspection fee + average outpatient treat fee + average registered fee + other outpatient fees	*yuan* per capita	Auxiliary

Continued

No.	Variable and SD equation (or value)	Unit	Variable type
66	outpatient service income = average outpatient service fee * outpatient number 0	ten thousand *yuan*	Auxiliary
67	average inpatient service fee＝average bed fee＋average inpatient inspection fee＋average inpatient surgery fee＋average inpatient treat fee＋ other hospitalization fees	*yuan* per capita	Auxiliary
68	inpatient service income＝average inpatient service fee * inpatient number 0	ten thousand *yuan*	Auxiliary
69	total medical income＝inpatient service income＋ outpatient service income	ten thousand *yuan*	Auxiliary
70	average medical expense for outpatient＝average outpatient drug fee＋average outpatient service fee	*yuan* per capita	Auxiliary
71	average medical expense for inpatient＝average hospitalization drug fee＋average inpatient service fee	*yuan* per capita	Auxiliary

6.3.2 Simulation without policy intervention

6.3.2.1 The income and expenditure of hospitals

Figure 6-7 presents the natural trends of hospital income and expenditure in 2010-2015 with the implementation of NEMS. It demonstrates that the hospital income and expenditure kept growing but the hospital net revenue shriank and even deficit occurred. This simulation result is consistent with the previous theoretical analysis. Hospital operation would be challenged if there is no effective compensation mechanism for primary health care facilities.

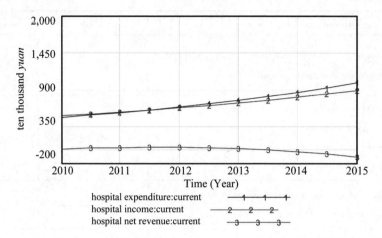

Figure 6-7　Trends of hospital income and expenditure under NEMS (2010-2015)

6.3.2.2　Medical expense of patients

Figure 6-8 illustrates a decreasing tendency of average drug fees per patient visit from 2010 to 2015. Instead of corresponding decline, the medical expense per patient increased (see Figure 6-9). However, the proportion of drug fee in medical expense reduced, as shown in Table 6-5.

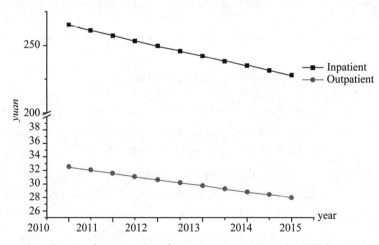

Figure 6-8　Trends of average drug fees per patient visit under NEMS (2010-2015)

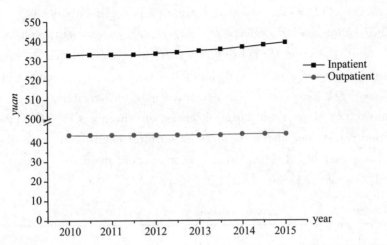

Figure 6-9　Trends of medical expense per patient visit under NEMS (2010-2015)

Table 6-5　The proportion of drug fee in medical expense for patients (2010-2015)

Time (year)	Drug fees (%) for inpatients	Drug fees (%) for outpatients
Initial	49. 76	74. 70
0. 5	49. 01	73. 64
1	48. 26	72. 55
1. 5	47. 51	71. 43
2	46. 76	70. 29
2. 5	46. 01	69. 12
3	45. 26	67. 92
3. 5	44. 51	66. 70
4	43. 76	65. 45
4. 5	43. 02	64. 18
Final	42. 28	62. 89

Selected Variables Runs: Current

6.3.3　Policy design and tentative assessment

Based on HO model, a series of policy experiments was designed to explore the feasible compensation methods for primary health settings. The experiments were made by altering key variables and parameters in the model.

6.3.3.1　Policy experiment I: increasing government subsidy

The compensation effect of increasing government subsidy was investigated by altering the subsidy rate (SR) in the HO model. All else being equal, we conducted a series of 7 simulation runs with an increment of 0.025 in SR (see Table 6-6), and then generated data on hospital net revenue and determined the impact on hospital operation. Figure 6-10 illustrates the simulation results and indicates that the hospital net revenue rose obviously with the increase of SR. Hospital net revenue could maintain a steady growth when SR reached 25% (see Line 5 in Figure 6-10).

Table 6-6　　　　　　Parameter values in policy experiment I

	current	sr1	sr2	sr3	sr4	sr5	sr6
SR	0.15	0.175	0.2	0.225	0.25	0.275	0.3

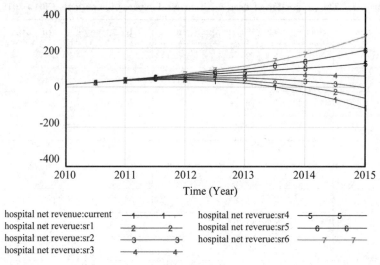

Figure 6-10　Trends of hospital net revenue by different government subsidy (2010-2015)

6.3.3.2　Policy experiment II: remuneration for pharmaceutical service

The remuneration for pharmaceutical service was spent on the dispensing activity as well as the professional service to help patients make the best use of their medicines. A fixed pharmaceutical service fee (PSF) was proposed for outpatients in prescriptions and for inpatients in times of medication advice. The PSF should be list separately when charged. Correspondingly, we added the PSF variables to the HO model. We assumed that outpatients got one prescription per visit and paid 2 *yuan* for PSF; inpatients got medication advice once a day and paid 4 *yuan* for PSF. The average length of stay (ALOS) is 9. 1 days according to the latest China Health Statistical Yearbook. Table 6-7 lists the supplemented variables and related SD equations for HO model.

Table 6-7　Variables and equations related to pharmaceutical service fee in HO model

No.	Variable and SD equation (or value)	Unit	Variable type
1	outpatient ps fee per time＝2	*yuan*	Constant
2	inpatient ps fee per time＝4	*yuan*	Constant
3	ALOS＝9. 1	day	Constant
4	outpatient ps fees＝outpatient ps fee per time * outpatient number	ten thousand *yuan*	Auxiliary
5	inpatient ps fee＝ALOS * inpatient ps fee per time	*yuan*	Auxiliary
6	inpatient ps fees＝inpatient ps fee * inpatient number	ten thousand *yuan*	Auxiliary
7	total ps income＝outpatient ps fees＋inpatient ps fees	ten thousand *yuan*	Auxiliary
8	hospital income ＝ government subsidy ＋ total drug income＋total medical income＋total other income＋total ps income	ten thousand *yuan*	Auxiliary
9	average medical expense for outpatient＝average outpatient drug fee＋average outpatient service fee＋outpatient ps fee per time	*yuan*	Auxiliary
10	average medical expense for inpatient ＝ average hospitalization drug fees ＋ average inpatient service fees＋inpatient ps fee	*yuan*	Auxiliary

The compensation effect of this proposed policy was then investigated by adjusting the conditions of remuneration as all else being equal. It was clear that the hospitals' deficit alleviated after paying for pharmaceutical service (see Figure 6-11). Then, we conducted 8 simulation runs with an increment of 1 in PSF (see Table 6-8), and generated data on hospital net revenues. Figure 6-12 illustrates the simulation results and indicates the descending of hospital net revenue slowed down with the increase of PSF. The downward trend was exactly reversed when 8 *yuan* per visit was charged for outpatient and 10 *yuan* per day was charged for inpatient (see Line 8 in Figure 6-12).

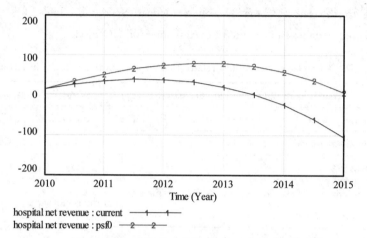

Figure 6-11　Trends of hospital net revenue with and without pharmaceutical service remuneration (2010-2015)

Table 6-8　　　　　Parameter values in policy experiment II

	current	psf0	psf1	psf2	psf3	psf4	psf5	psf6	psf7	psf8
PSF (outpatient)	0	2	3	4	5	6	7	8	9	10
PSF (inpatient)	0	4	5	6	7	8	9	10	11	12

To further investigate the amount of remuneration, we conducted another five simulation runs with an interval of 1 *yuan* around 8 *yuan* for inpatient and 10 *yuan* for inpatient. The hospital net revenue could also maintain stable growth when PSF was 7 *yuan* for outpatient and 12 *yuan* for inpatient or 9 *yuan* for both inpatient and outpatient (see Table 6-9).

At the beginning of paying for pharmaceutical service, the average medical expense for patients increased by about 15%-20%. However, the gap of medical expense before and after the intervention narrowed over time, as shown in Figure 6-13 and Figure 6-14. Therefore, the remuneration for pharmaceutical service was considered rational and may refer to 7-9 *yuan* per visit for outpatient service and 9-12 *yuan* per day for inpatient service.

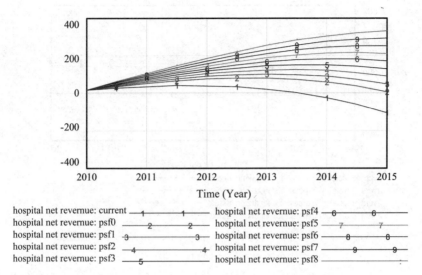

Figure 6-12　Trends of hospital net revenue by different pharmaceutical
service remuneration (2010-2015)

**Table 6-9　Trends of hospital net revenue by different pharmaceutical
service remuneration (2010-2015)**

Time (Year)	Pharmaceutical service fee (outpatient, inpatient) *yuan*						
	0, 0 (current)	8, 10 (psf6)	7, 10 (psf6a)	7, 11 (psf6b)	7, 12 (psf6c)	8, 9 (psf6d)	9, 9 (psf6e)
Initial	14.11	14.11	14.11	14.11	14.11	14.11	14.11
0.5	26.17	53.52	51.31	52.27	53.23	52.56	54.77
1	34.54	90.77	86.26	88.28	90.29	88.75	93.26
1.5	38.72	125.46	118.58	121.75	124.92	122.29	129.17
2	38.15	157.15	147.81	152.25	156.68	152.71	162.05
2.5	32.21	185.34	173.47	179.29	185.10	179.52	191.39
3	20.19	209.47	194.98	202.31	209.64	202.14	216.64
3.5	1.31	228.91	211.70	220.69	229.68	219.92	237.13
4	−25.32	242.92	222.90	233.71	244.51	232.11	252.13
4.5	−60.67	250.70	227.78	240.57	253.37	237.91	260.83
Final	−105.87	251.34	225.41	240.38	255.36	236.37	262.30

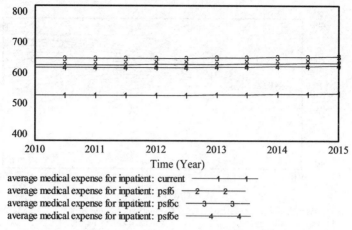

Figure 6-13　Average medical expense for inpatient by different pharmaceutical service fee (2010-2015)

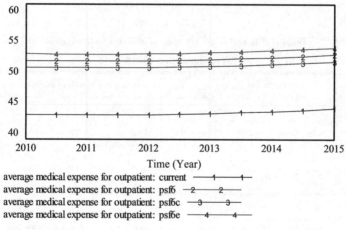

Figure 6-14　Average medical expense for outpatient by different pharmaceutical service fee (2010-2015)

6.3.3.3　Policy experiment Ⅲ: improving medical service pricing

The compensation effect of improving medical service pricing was investigated by altering the values of increase rate of medical service fee (IRMSF) in the HO model. A series of 6 simulation runs was conducted with an increase of 50% each time (see Table 6-10) to generate the data on hospital net revenue (see Figure 6-15). It can be seen that the hospital net revenue was growing steadily when IRMSF increased by 1.5 times (see Line 4 in Figure

6-15). In this case, the IRMSF was 21% for outpatient and 9% for inpatient. Also, the medical expense of patients increased correspondingly (see Figure 6-16 and Figure 6-17).

Table 6-10   **Parameter values in policy experiment III**

	current	msf1	msf2	msf3	msf4	msf5	msf6
IRMSF (outpatient)	0. 0843	0. 1265	0. 1686	0. 2108	0. 2529	0. 2951	0. 3372
IRMSF (inpatient)	0. 036	0. 054	0. 072	0. 09	0. 108	0. 126	0. 144

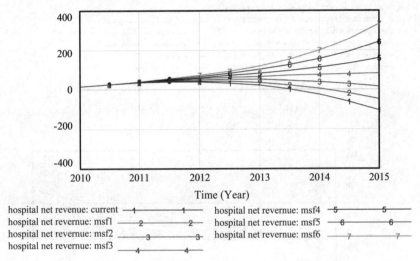

Figure 6-15　Trends of hospital net revenue by different

medical service pricing (2010-2015)

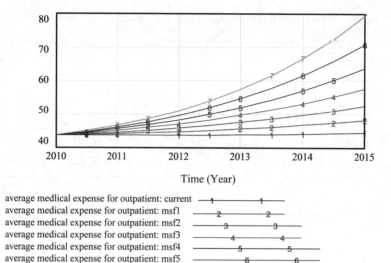

average medical expense for outpatient: current
average medical expense for outpatient: msf1
average medical expense for outpatient: msf2
average medical expense for outpatient: msf3
average medical expense for outpatient: msf4
average medical expense for outpatient: msf5
average medical expense for outpatient: msf6

Figure 6-16　Trends of average medical expense for outpatients by
different medical service pricing（2010-2015）

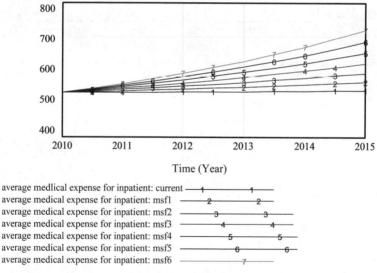

average medical expense for inpatient: current
average medical expense for inpatient: msf1
average medical expense for inpatient: msf2
average medical expense for inpatient: msf3
average medical expense for inpatient: msf4
average medical expense for inpatient: msf5
average medical expense for inpatient: msf6

Figure 6-17　Trends of average medical expense for inpatients by
different medical service pricing（2010-2015）

6. 3. 3. 4　Policy experiment IV: combined compensation mechanism

Meanwhile, we explored the compensation effect of a combined compensation mechanism, which was a synthesis of the above three methods. Due to the pool efforts, each parameter in this experiment can be with a milder adjustment compared to the previous tests. Totally we made 5 simulation runs. The PSF was adjusted as 2-6 *yuan* for outpatients and as 4-8 *yuan* for inpatients and the step value for both was 1 *yuan*. SR was adjusted as 0. 15-0. 225 with an increase of 10% each time. The IRMSF was adjusted as 0. 0843-0. 1265 for outpatients and as 0. 036-0. 054 for inpatients, also with an increase of 10% each time. Table 6-10 lists the values of these parameters in each simulation.

The simulation results are illustrated in Figure 6-18. It is clear that the hospital net revenue was able to keep growing when the cc3 compensation mechanism was adopted (see Line 4 in Figure 6-18). In this case, each parameter increased by about 30% compared to the initial value. The medical expense per patient visit increased by an average of 11% (see Table 6-12). However, the proportion of drug fee in medical expense further declined compared with the simulation results without intervention by about 10% (see Table 6-13).

Table 6-11　　　　**Parameter values in policy experiment IV**

	current	cc1	cc2	cc3	cc4	cc5
SR	0. 15	0. 165	0. 18	0. 195	0. 21	0. 225
PSF (outpatient)	0	2	3	4	5	6
PSF (inpatient)	0	4	5	6	7	8
IRMSF (outpatient)	0. 0843	0. 0927	0. 1012	0. 1096	0. 1180	0. 1265
IRMSF (inpatient)	0. 0360	0. 0396	0. 0432	0. 0468	0. 0504	0. 0540

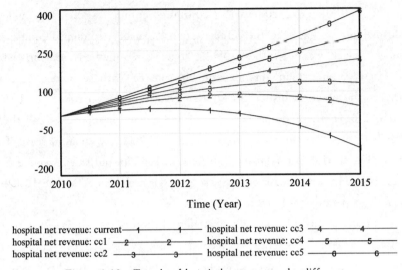

hospital net revenue: current ——1—— 1—— hospital net revenue: cc3 ——4—— 4——
hospital net revenue: cc1 ——2—— 2—— hospital net revenue: cc4 ——5—— 5——
hospital net revenue: cc2 ——3—— 3—— hospital net revenue: cc5 ——6—— 6——

Figure 6-18   Trends of hospital net revenue by different
compensation behavior（2010-2015）

Table 6-12   Trends of average medical expense per patient visit under cc3
compensation mechanism（2010-2015）

Time (Year)	average medical expense for inpatient (*yuan*)		Difference (%)	average medical expense for outpatient (*yuan*)		Difference (%)
	current	cc3		current	cc3	
Initial	532.82	587.42	10.25	43.59	47.59	9.18
0.5	532.85	588.65	10.47	43.55	47.69	9.50
1	533.02	590.07	10.70	43.54	47.83	9.84
1.5	533.31	591.67	10.94	43.56	48.01	10.21
2	533.74	593.46	11.19	43.61	48.23	10.61
2.5	534.30	595.43	11.44	43.68	48.50	11.03
3	535.00	597.59	11.70	43.78	48.82	11.49
3.5	535.83	599.95	11.97	43.92	49.18	11.98
4	536.79	602.50	12.24	44.08	49.59	12.50
4.5	537.89	605.25	12.52	44.28	50.06	13.06
Final	539.13	608.19	12.81	44.51	50.59	13.66

Table 6-13   The proportion of drug fee in medical expense under cc3
compensation mechanism (2010-2015)

Time (Year)	drug fees (%) for inpatients	drug fees (%) for outpatients
Initial	45.13	68.42
0.5	44.36	67.25
1	43.59	66.05
1.5	42.82	64.81
2	42.05	63.55
2.5	41.28	62.25
3	40.52	60.92
3.5	39.75	59.56
4	38.99	58.18
4.5	38.23	56.77
Final	37.48	55.34

Selected Variables Runs: cc3

6.4 Discussion

6.4.1 Medicine availability

Our findings indicates that the amount of medicines in PHCs decreased after NEMS implementation. This might be affected by the policy that only essential medicines were allowed in public primary health settings. So in this case, a key point was to ensure the high availability of essential medicines. Based on the monitoring data from the regions, the availability of essential medicines was 66.83% in PHCs. A survey in 2007 showed that pharmacies in Shandong primary care hospitals supplied a median of 26% of the WMs and 25% of the TCMs on the NEML and in Gansu the figures were lower at 19% and 33% respectively. (Chen et al., 2010) By contrast, the availability of essential medicines was improved. Also, this research result is higher than that reported in over 40 low- and middle-income countries (44%) in 2011. (WHO, 2011b)

Furthermore, the availability is associated with the efficiency of medicine delivery. In our survey, the average response rate of delivery was close to 100%; however the arrival rate of medicines was only 86.45%. This might create medicine shortage in PHCs, which may force patients to purchase from private sector, where prices were generally higher, and thereby had a negative effect on ATM. The problems in drug supply had not only influenced service quality and clinic revenue but also led to a misperception among patients that the doctors were unwilling to provide care that was not profitable. (Li et al., 2013)

6.4.2　Hospital operation

The findings shows an increasing tendency in the number of patient visits at PHCs after the introduction of NEMS. The decrease in drug prices and more rational drug prescribing might have contributed to the increased uptake of health services, because drugs prescribed from major hospitals are more expensive due to the ability of hospitals to have margins of up to 30%, whereas primary institutions must sell at cost. (Yang et al., 2012) Also, the improvements in rural health insurance might be a contributor.

The hospital income has increased by 24.26% between 2009 and 2011. However, the hospital net revenue declined and a loss of 21.79 thousand *yuan* occurred in 2011. This founding is consistent with other researches in China (Chen et al., 2012; Song & Bian, 2013c). A plenty of studies have revealed that the decrease of the net revenue is mainly due to the government subsidy (Wang, Zheng, Qu & Liu, 2011; Zhu, Wang & Jiang, 2012). According to the old drug policy, public hospitals were allowed to mark up the medicine prices by 15%. (Song & Bian, 2011a) So, most local governments simply calculated the subsidy as 15% of their drug revenue. However, the actual drug markup was much higher than 15%. Also, the HO simulation result shows that the hospital net revenue kept shrinking if there was no policy intervention. The substantial profit loss may result in shortage in routine operational activities, sales of diagnostics, technologies, or other revenue generation methods to cover basic operational costs, and weak ability to maintain the essential medicine system. (Song & Bian, 2011b) Therefore, sustainable mechanisms to compensate primary health care facilities are critically wanted. In addition, the results show the structure of hospital income was changed and the proportion of drug income declined. It indicates the incentive of hospital generating profits from medicines is being changed by the NEMS.

6. 4. 3　Compensation of zero-profit policy

The findings of the tentative experiments show all the four proposed methods are feasible. Among them, the combined compensation mechanism can achieve the better effect with milder adjustment and is an optimal choice. Also, it is the most popular mode in the current pilot programs. The joint measures identified for the comprehensive compensation include: increasing government subsidy by 19. 5% a year; charging PSF 4 *yuan* per prescription for outpatients and 6 *yuan* per day for inpatients; and improving prices of out-patient services by 10. 96%, in-patient services by 4. 68% annually. Under this mechanism, the remuneration of pharmaceutical services can be considered to be covered by health insurance schemes. In addition, the improvement of medical service prices is not a simple behavior of price increase. Hospitals should be encouraged to improve the quality and efficiency of health services and thereby improve the relative prices.

6. 4. 4　HO model used in this study

Most applications of System Dynamics have addressed issue-specific problems or sector specific issues in health system, including the dynamics of human services delivery, diffusion of new medical technologies, management of acute or chronic diseases, patient flows, and so on. The HO model used in this study is an initial simplified SD representation in hospital income and expenditure. The results of this study proves that the HO model can quantitatively simulate the structure and behaviors of the real hospital operational system and would be broadened to a simulation platform for policy research. At a macroscopic level, it can be used to assess a variety of hospital compensation mechanisms put forward during the reform progress. And at a microscopic level, it might be applied to a specific hospital as a decision-making tool in daily operation.

6. 5 Summary

NEMS has improved the availability of essential medicines and increased the uptake of health services in PHCs. Also, the structure of hospital income has been changed and the proportion of drug income declined. However, most primary health-care facilities encountered substantial financial losses. Based on a simple and reliable HO model, a combined compensation mechanism is put forward in this study, which is considered as an optimal choice at present.

Chapter 7   Awareness, perception and satisfaction among stakeholders

To date, the first three-year implementation plan of NEMS has been completed. The effects of its introduction in China are being widely investigated. However, little information is focused on people's responses to essential medicines. Clearly, there is a need to investigate the residents and the professionals' views as they are the direct demanders and providers of essential medicines and this knowledge will aid in further improving the implementation of NEMS. Consequently, the purpose of this chapter is to explore the awareness, perception and satisfaction related to NEMS among these stakeholders and to provide the baseline data for policy improvement.

7. 1   Materials and method

7. 1. 1   Study setting

A questionnaire survey was conducted in 16 PHCs in Ningxia Province. Ningxia is located in Western China and is at a low economic level. There are many people living in a very lower-quality life especially in the south mountain area and encountering serious problems of difficult and costly access to health care services. The feedback in this place could be an important indicator for measuring the quality of the new NEMS.

7. 1. 2   Subjects

Two groups of participants were randomly enrolled in this study: rural residents and primary health workers (PHWs). A total of 15 residents and 10 PHWs were supposed to be surveyed from different hospitals. However, due to the limited conditions in the sites during the survey period, only 178 questionnaires were distributed to the residents and 134 were distributed to the PHWs. 3 rural residents failed to provide complete information, leaving a total of 309 valid sets of responses. The response rate is 99.04%. The identities of all participants were kept blind and all were specifically informed that they were free to refuse to participate in the study or withdraw at any moment during the study. Written informed consents were obtained from the participants before the questionnaire survey.

7.1.3 Instrument

Two self-compiled questionnaires were used in the survey: one was for rural residents (see Appendix III), and the other was for PHWs (see Appendix IV). Both questionnaires consists of four parts. The first part contains sociodemographic questions i.e. age, gender, level of education, income, et al. The second part assesses their awareness with NEMS. The third part is about their perceptions on the changes brought by NEMS and the last part assesses their satisfaction with NEMS. Additionally, at the end of the two questionnaires, an open-ended question is conducted to further investigate their medicine demands.

The answers to most questions were measured on a 5-point Likert Scale with the lowest response on the one end of the score and the highest response on the highest score on the scale. Finally, the general satisfaction was evaluated on a 10-point scale, with 0 representing very unsatisfied and 10 representing very satisfied.

7.1.4 Data analysis

All analyses were entered into the EpiData software 3.1 and were analyzed using SPSS 19.0. Category data were analyzed for frequency distribution and percentage of subjects; Quantitative data were analyzed by mean and standard deviation (Sd) value. The general satisfaction was defined as below: > 8.5, absolutely satisfied; 6.5-8.5, quite satisfied; 4.5-6.5, relative satisfied; 2.5-4.5, dissatisfied; and <2.5, very dissatisfied. The final score for satisfaction was expressed as a rate and the formulation was: the overall satisfaction rate＝(No. of absolutely satisfied＋No. of quite satisfied＋ No. of relative satisfied)/ the total number of subjects ＊ 100％. In addition, a multiple linear regression was employed to explore the influence factors of satisfaction score: the dependent variable was the general satisfaction score of each respondent; the independent variables included gender, age, education, income, knowledge on NEMS, and so on.

7. 2　Results

7. 2. 1　Demographic characteristics of the study participants

A total of 175 rural residents and 134 PHWs were studied of the rural residents who responded, the mean age was 41. 23 (Sd＝13. 18), with half being male (50. 3％). Most of them are with middle school or lower education (88. 6％). The majority of them (94. 3％) were insured by New Rural Cooperative Medical Scheme. Of the 134 PHWs, the age range was 18-61 years old (mean 35. 43, Sd ＝ 8. 934). By gender, female health workers contributed 57. 5％ with the male to female ratio of 0. 8:1. Most of them are junior college graduates (64. 2％) and the mean length of employment is 12. 4 (Sd＝9. 29) years. The profile of questionnaire respondents is summarized in Table 7-1.

Table 7-1　　　Demographic characteristic of study participants

Characteristics	Rural residents		Health workers	
	N	％	N	％
Total	175	100	134	100
Gender				
Male	88	50. 3	57	42. 5
Female	87	49. 7	77	57. 5
Age (years)				
＜30	32	18. 3	30	22. 4
30-50	99	56. 6	94	70. 1
＞50	44	25. 1	10	7. 5

Continued

Education level				
High school and below	170	97. 1	24	17. 9
Junior college	3	1. 7	86	64. 2
Bachelor	2	1. 1	24	17. 9
Length of employment (years)				
<5	—	—	33	24. 6
5-10	—	—	31	23. 1
11-20	—	—	47	35. 1
>20	—	—	23	17. 2
Professional qualification				
NA	—	—	30	22. 4
Primary	—	—	72	53. 7
Junior	—	—	30	22. 4
Senior	—	—	2	1. 5
Working category				
Physician	—	—	76	56. 7
Pharmacist	—	—	19	14. 2
Nursing staff	—	—	21	15. 7
Laboratory technician	—	—	7	5. 2
Management staff	—	—	11	8. 2
Monthly income (*yuan*)				
<1000	—	—	22	16. 4
1000-2000	—	—	67	50
>2000	—	—	45	33. 6
Household income per month (*yuan*)				
<1000	118	67. 4	—	—
1000-2000	36	20. 6	—	—
>2000	21	12	—	—

7. 2. 2　The residents' view on NEMS

Generally, 138 (78.9%) residents had no idea of NEMS. Only 19 (10.9%) showed familiar or relative familiar and nobody was quite familiar with NEMS. In addition, 134 (76.6%) of the residents did not know that essential medicines were sold at procurement cost in PHCs. And 26 (14.9%) heard of this zero-profit policy but did not know the details. Only 15 (8.5%) were familiar or relatively familiar with the zero-profit policy. As for the reimbursement policy of essential medicines, 86 (49.1%) were familiar or relatively familiar. However, 71 (40.6%) still had no idea of it.

Regarding the medicine price, 82 (46.8%) of the 175 responded residents felt that it decreased or greatly decreased after NEMS implementation. However, 80 (45.7%) thought there was no change and 13 (7.5%) felt that the price increased. Nevertheless, most residents (86.3%) were satisfied or very satisfied with the current price level. Only 21 (12.0%) felt dissatisfied and 3 (1.7%) were very dissatisfied. Regarding the medical costs, a total of 95 (54.3%) perceived that the total medical expenses per visit reduced or greatly reduced in the post-implementation period of NEMS. However, 11 (6.3%) felt that the total medical expenses increased. Furthermore, a total of 134 (76.6%) residents were satisfied or very satisfied with the quality of essential medicines. But regarding the quantity of essential medicines, more than half (52.6%) perceived the current amounts could not satisfy their medicine demands. The medicines they proposed to supplement included (list by the frequency of the occurrence): cold medicine, gynecology medicine, cardiovascular medicine, nutrition medicine (i.e. health care products, Vitamin, cod liver oil), anti-inflammatory medicine, pediatric medicine, and so on. In addition, 116 (66.3%) of residents perceived an improvement of the pharmaceutical service in hospitals. A high proportion (96%) of respondents felt satisfied or very satisfied with the current medicine dispensing activity. As for the professional services to help making the best use of medicines, the overall percentage of residents who were satisfied or very satisfied was 96.6%.

The final satisfaction score among the surveyed residents ranged between 2 and 10 with an average of 7.16 (Sd = 1.86), indicating that the rural residents were quite satisfied with NEMS. The overall satisfaction rate was 93.31%. And based on multivariable linear regression analysis, the general satisfaction of the residents was independently associated with their knowledge on reimbursement policy ($p=0.009$, OR$=0.317$, 95% CI: 0.08-0.554).

7.2.3 The health workers' view on NEMS

Acquired responses reveals that 131 (97.8%) of the health professionals were familiar or very familiar with the NEMS program. Furthermore, the majority of them (97.1%) had an idea of EML. Specifically, 16 (11.9%) felt very familiar; 72 (53.7%) were familiar; and 41 (30.6%) were relatively familiar. In the past two years, 46.3% of the health workers received the training on NEMS. Most of them were trained for once or twice (see Table 7-2). However, all the PHWs in the survey expected to get more trainings.

Table 7-2   The frequency of trainings about NEMS on primary health workers

Training times	No. of respondents	%
0	72	53.7
1	23	17.2
2	20	14.9
3	7	5.2
≥4	12	8.8
Total	134	100

A total of 132 (98.5%) health workers were satisfied or very satisfied with the pricing of essential medicines. And 123 (91.8%) were satisfied or very satisfied with the quality of essential medicines. Regarding the effects of essential medicines, 48 (35.8%) of the respondents felt that they were equivalent to those of other medicines. However, 41 (30.6%) thought the effects of essential medicines tended to be a little worse. Also, the majority of the health workers (81.4%) perceived the amount of essential medicines could not satisfy their clinical needs. The medicines they were proposed to supplement contained (list by the frequency of the occurrence): gynecology medicine, cardiovascular medicine, pediatric medicine, digestive and stomachic medicine, emergency medicine, antibiotics, cold medicine, rheumatism medicine, and so on. After the implementation of NEMS, about

42 (31. 3%) PHWs perceived that their department income reduced. Still most (66, 49. 3%) health workers thought there was no difference. Also, the majority of them (80. 6%) reported that there was no change in their personal incomes.

Generally, almost 90% of PHWs expected to promote NEMS nationwide. The final satisfaction score among professionals ranged between 2 and 10 with an average of 6. 93 (Sd=1. 91), indicating that the health professionals who responded to this survey were quite satisfied with NEMS. The overall satisfaction rate was 92. 54%. In multivariable linear regression analysis, the general satisfaction of professionals was independently associated with their knowledge on NEMS (p=0. 03, OR=0. 663, 95% CI: 0. 234-1. 092).

7. 3 Discussion

The samples in this questionnaire are limited to the subjects in Ningxia. Thus, the generalization of the findings needs to be treated with caution. However, Ningxia is the front runner of China's NEMS as well as a representative of the under-developed areas. So the results might be a reflection of China's reform progress and are useful to developing nations in advocating for the incorporation of effective NEMS.

7. 3. 1 Awareness

The findings of the survey shows that the rural residents in Ningxia had a low awareness of NEMS. Although some of them heard of the policies related to NEMS, most of them only knew the name but did not know the specific contents, let alone the significance of promoting NEMS. Other researches in China also have the same findings. For instance, a survey in Nanjing shows that less than one fifth of the rural residents heard of NEMS and most had no awareness of it. (Huang et al., 2011) Rural residents with lower education level and less household income always have poor access to health care and are the targeted population of NEMS. However, due to the low awareness, they might not understand the importance of NEMS, which leads to the low recognition of essential medicines and hinders the full potential of essential medicines. Thus, it is necessary to enhance the propaganda to the rural residents through a variety of ways. A poster competition in community has proved extremely successful to raise public awareness in Indonesia. (Husniah, 2005)

Fortunately, the findings indicate the PHWs in this area had certain awareness with NEMS. The majority of them were familiar or very familiar with NEMS and EML. Compared with a western province where 63.7% of the population were reported to have an idea of NEMS (Yan et al., 2010), the PHWs in Ningxia had a high awareness. In addition, the result of this research indicates there was lack of a normal and systematic training mechanism. Although 46.3% of the participants had received the training on NEMS, however most of them were only trained once or twice during the past two years. Most participants expect to get more trainings.

7.3.2 Perception and satisfaction

The stakeholders' satisfaction in this study mainly came considered from their perceptions on the price, quality and quantity of essential medicines. Furthermore, a close eye was kept on residents' perceptions on the total medical expenses and the pharmaceutical services in the hospital. Also, the PHWs' attitudes on the changes of their personal and department incomes were taken into account.

Firstly, the majority of the residents and PHWs was found satisfied or very satisfied with the price and the quality of essential medicines. Most residents had perceived a decrease in drug prices. The result presented here reinforces the conclusions in Chapter 4. However, both residents and professionals perceived that the quantity of essential medicines was not enough, which is consistent with many previous researches in China. Many factors may contribute to the unmet demand of medicines. The poor selection of essential medicines might be a dominant contributor. A study in three rural counties in western China reports that about 1/3 of the drugs in common use by the local people cannot be found in the list, and 1/3 drugs on the list were rarely used. The medicine use habit was another important factor. (Song & Bian, 2013b) After NEMS, only essential medicines were allowed to stock in primary care facilities. Neither physicians nor patients have adapted to the new medication pattern. Also, the inefficient distribution might contribute to the dissatisfaction due to the low medicine profit and high transportation cost in this process especially for the remote rural areas. Acquired responses from both sides suggest the necessity of supplementing more gynecology medicine, cardiovascular medicine, pediatric medicine, antibiotics and cold medicine to EML.

Next, the findings indicate that the residents felt a decrease in their total medical expenses. The observed decreases in drug prices and the more rational prescribing might be major contributors. In many developing countries, medicines constitute the largest household health expenditure. By focusing pharmaceutical expenditure on essential drugs, the cost-effectiveness of government and out-of-pocket drug expenditure can be enhanced and health impact heightened. (WHO, 2000) Meanwhile, most PHWs have not felt the changes in their personal or department income. However, still one third of the PHWs perceived their department incomes decreased. The hospitals would deal with greater numbers of patients in the post-implementation period of NEMS. It is essential to ensure a sustainable financial compensation for hospitals to ensure their routine operational activities and the high quality of health services.

Finally, the results indicate NEMS had been welcomed by stakeholders and the overall satisfaction rate was over 90%. Moreover, the residents with better knowledge on reimbursement policy and the PHWs with better knowledge on NEMS showed a higher satisfaction with NEMS. This finding is a practical use of the Knowledge-Attitude-Practice theory. The sufficient information on NEMS can gradually build the social trust in essential medicines, thereby reducing the demands for the drugs which will not bring additional health benefits. Also, this finding indicates the rural residents were more concerned with the out-pocket expenditure in the essential medicine reform.

7.4 Summary

In conclusion, this study identifies a high satisfaction among the stakeholders towards NEMS, which is a reflection of the developments in health system. However, a close eye must be kept on the low awareness of rural residents on NEMS, which might weaken their recognition on essential medicines and hinder the policy implementation. Therefore, further considerations should be given on public education program. Also, efforts are still made to improve the selection and delivery of essential medicines and to ensure sustainable compensation mechanisms for health care providers.

Chapter 8   Conclusion and policy recommendation

8. 1   Conclusion

This study summarizes the recent attempts of China's NEMS and establishes a framework for evaluation, It helps to assess the main features of NEMS midway through China's health-sector reform during 2009-2011 and has found a mixture of benefits as well as challenges to the system's sustainability. It is concluded that NEMS mostly heads towards the right direction and has its intended impact on containment of drug prices and more appropriate use of medications. The comprehensive approach of China's NEMS could be an excellent example of adaptation of the WHO essential medicine concept, which is informative for other countries.

8. 1. 1   Achievements and gaps in the policy objectives

Regional experiences reported in the present study confirm that a great deal of progress has been achieved within such a short time frame. A median decrease of 34. 38% in price was witnessed between 2009 and 2010. Particularly, the largest price decline was observed for anti-inflammatory and cardiovascular drugs. The declines were also recorded in the mean number of drugs prescribed per patient and the proportion of patients being prescribed antibiotics. Increases in the utilization of essential medicines have occurred. The injection and hormone use were improved significantly. The observed decrease in drug prices together with more rational drug prescribing led to increased uptake of health services. The availability of essential medicines reached 66. 83% in PHCs, where the structure of hospital income has been changed and the proportion of drug income decreased. A high satisfaction was expressed by stakeholders and the overall satisfaction rate towards NEMS was over 90%.

Although some breakthroughs have been achieved, daunting challenges and issues persist. The medicine prices remained high compared to international reference prices. Medicines were often unaffordable for poor residents. The new shortages of some drugs occurred. Over-prescription of antibiotics and injections as well as polypharmacy remained common compared to WHO standards. Importantly, most primary health-care facilities encountered substantial financial losses. The compensation of health-care providers for NEMS-related reductions had been largely ineffective.

8. 1. 2 Difficulties and challenges in the implementation

The poor outcomes of the essential medicines programme might be indicative of problems in programme design and implementation and further analyses are required to address remaining difficulties and challenges to bring about the reform goals.

Firstly, the current official documents for this reform provide only guiding principles that encourage the local adaptation and piloting of the NEMS, including the use of the EML and strategies to compensate health care providers for income lost as a result of the zero profit policy. More complete implementation of policies is still needed from the national level. The lack of specific policies has caused poor performability in the implementation.

Secondly, selection of medicines for both the national and provincial lists is not clearly based on cost-effectiveness. Under a poorly regulated system, an important issue is what influence the pharmaceutical industry might be exerting on drug selection.

Thirdly, the recommended two-envelop procurement procedures have adversely affected the supply of some essential medicines. In view of the poor qualifying competition of technical specifications, competitive bidding on prices has meant "the winning death" (the production of some essential drugs by some manufacturers ceased because the biding severely curtailed the profit to be made by manufacturers) or that manufacturers producing inferior medicines have won some bids. In addition, widespread corruption (kickbacks to providers) persists in the procurement process. Thus, despite the zero-profit policy, income for health-care providers is still not separated from drug prescription.

Fourthly, the zero-profit policy aims to compress the profit space of the supply chain and improve the medicine affordability. However, it could also result in more opportunist behaviors of the manufacturers, distributors and health-care providers due to the loss of vested interests. Especially, there are problems with how the compensation to health-care providers is calculated. The compensation based on previous practice still encourages doctors to over-prescribe and, when faced with several options, to prescribe the most expensive drug. Also, the hospital compensation is challenged by financing. Local governments are expected to contribute two thirds of new government funding, and in poor areas they might not have the means to do so or might shift funds from other social needs.

Fifthly, due to the limited number of essential medicines, the exclusive usage policy in primary health-care settings might influence the distribution of service contacts between township- and county-level providers and undermine China's attempt to provide access to primary health care. Furthermore, the poor recognition of essential medicines leads to the lack of demand and often causes conflicts between the prescription of doctors and the medical needs of patients. Public knowledge and acceptance of generics, essential medicines, and rational use are critical to the success of the essential medicines reform.

8.2 Policy recommendation

The solutions for the remaining challenges are analyzed within the framework of the popularly used drug management cycle (DMC) approach, as shown in Figure 8-1. Drug management functions are always undertaken in four principal phases, which are interlinked and are reinforced by appropriate management support systems. From drug selection to drug use, passing through procurement, storage and distribution, a whole range of management measures are required within a given legal and policy context. Within this framework, four targeted recommendations have been proposed for the further improvement of China's NEMS.

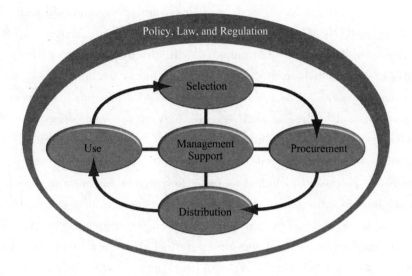

Figure 8-1　Drug management cycle (MSH/WHO, 1997)

8. 2. 1　Selection of essential medicines

The selection of essential medicines is the core of NEMS and also a key issue that causes social discontent. The process of selection should be based on the highest quality scientific evidence, evidence-based clinical treatment guidelines, and careful consideration of population health needs. A standing committee should be appointed to give technical advice. The committee may be composed of experts in all spheres of medical and pharmaceutical practice, including clinical pharmacists and pharmacologists, medical specialists, pediatricians, nurses, public health workers, and health workers at grass-roots level. Consultations may be organized with interested parties, including representatives of professional bodies, pharmaceutical manufacturers, consumer organizations and the government budget and finance group. Policies should be made to provide technical support to provinces, especially to undeveloped provinces which might not be able to carry out evidence-based selection. Local levels should dynamically monitor the use of essential drugs and provide swift feedback in order to make reasonable adjustments for EML. The feedback from this research suggests increasing gynecological medicines, cardiovascular medicines, pediatric medicines, antibiotics and cold medicines.

The latest NEML (2012 edition) was released on March 15, 2013, effective as of May 1, 2013. Compared with the previous version, the new NEML has expanded from 307 to 502 products, including 317 western medicines and 203 TCMs. Also, the new NEML expands its coverage of diseases. Specialty drugs, such as oncology drugs and drugs for blood diseases, are listed in it. For the first time, human insulin products are included as well. Moreover, nearly 200 drugs in the new NEML can be used for pediatric purposes, including all pediatric vaccines currently in the Chinese national immunization plan. In addition, the amount of foreign drugs is obviously increased; even some of blockbuster products from notable multinational pharmaceutical companies are included, such as Plavix (Sanofi/ BMS), Glucobay (Bayer), Norvasc (Pfizer) and Diovan (Novartis). In the previous list, only Zocor from Merck is included.

8.2.2 Procurement and supply

The essential medicine system created a desirable market share for which manufacturers would compete. (Charles & Lu, 2011) Given the anticipated intensive competition, a well-regulated bidding procurement system is firstly required. Firstly, the key point is to adopt stronger and more uniform criteria to accurately capture product quality and firm performance in technical biding. The quality and safety of medicines must be assured prior to the evaluation of a commercial bid. Where the price of medicines in commercial biding is obviously low, an in-depth comprehensive assessment should be made in order to avoid the vicious competition. Additionally, the competitive bidding on prices in the current tendering system can be replaced by cost-effectiveness evaluation if applicable. The incremental cost-effectiveness ratio (ICER) can be considered as a proxy variable during evaluation. Secondly, regarding the distribution, it is attemptable to explore innovative ways to ensure the supply. For example, medicines can be delivered with the aid of logistics services (such as postal service) which can provide wide coverage in China. DHL has partnered with UNICEF Kenya to reduce childhood mortality in Kenya by providing logistics expertise, in-kind donations and technical support to improve the medical supply chain. (Kyla, Lois & Orin, 2011) Furthermore, for those in charge of rural remote areas, we may also consider providing a special offer through fiscal means (such as tax deduction and exemption) or monetary means (such as commercial credit). Thirdly, the government can carry out designated production within a certain scope, especially for the low-profit but high-efficacy drugs as well as the orphan drugs, to avoid the stock out. Fourthly, it is important to strengthen the scientific supervision and regulation in procurement and distribution process. The penalties for manufacturers, who are unable to comply with the contracts, should be introduced. The side-benefits of such measures may be a much-needed consolidation and better regulation of China's pharmaceutical industry. In short, it is essential to establish a public-private mixed medicine supply system. Under this system, the role of the government is to maintain strict regulation of the pharmaceutical sector to prevent and punish opportunistic behavior. And the establishment of distribution relationship is handled by the market mechanisms which permit competition. The examples of efficient drug supply systems have existed in some countries in Africa, Asia, Latin America and elsewhere in the world and is recommended by WHO. (Quick et al., 2002)

8. 2. 3　Compensation for zero-profit policy

International experience reveals the zero-markup rate policy for drugs is not isolated and should be combined with government budgetary management and separation of revenue and expenditure accounts. Each province should coordinate the use of the fiscal subsidy and support the poor regions through an increase in payment transfer. In localities where necessary conditions are satisfied, revenue and expenditure can be separated. However, it is a difficult task for governments to take the entire responsibility to fill the income gap. Government-supervised multiple compensation mechanisms can work together to broaden the channels of compensation. In spite of the government subsidy, the first step is to give full play to medical insurance. Various medical insurance payments, such as capitation and diagnosis-related groups, should be carried out to effectively utilize medical resources and control medical expenditures. Next, the prices of medical services should be raised appropriately, while revenue from large kinds of equipment and medical consumables should be reduced. A fixed pharmaceutical service fee can be introduced. Also, non-governmental investments should be utilized.

(Charles & Lu, 2011) Our findings suggest increasing government subsidy by 19. 5% a year, charging pharmaceutical service fee 4 *yuan* per prescription for outpatients and 6 *yuan* per day for inpatients, and improving prices of out-patient services by 10. 96%, in patient services by 4. 68% annually.

8. 2. 4　Usage of essential medicines

The priority use of essential medicines is worth advocating. However, doctors in primary health-care institutions should not be limited to prescribing only essential medicines and should enjoy some autonomous rights within a certain range. WHO has recommended to consider establishing an administrative or budgetary "safety valve" for the limited supply and use of non-listed medicines. (WHO, 2002b) In China, the government can consider setting a safety line based on sales revenue. For example, the sales of non-listed medicines should be no more than 10% of the total. Another important issue is to facilitate the implementation of evidence-based treatment guidelines and essential medicine formulary and directly target all key stakeholders, in order to guide clinical care and prescribing practices, improve the authority of the EML as well as to enhance the medication convergence. Health delivery systems should routinely assess drug use and adopt policies or ongoing quality improvement programs to promote appropriate drug use. Besides, the concept of essential medicine should be incorporated into the basic education and continuing education of health workers. Economic incentives can be used to foster pharmacists' selling of essential drugs. The PBS model in Australian has provided a good reference. Also, it is necessary to strengthen the patient and consumer education to make them understand and trust essential medicines and gradually change the bias that essential medicines are second rate medicines for poor people, thereby reducing their demand for the drugs which will not bring additional health benefits.

References

Babar, Z. U., Ibrahim, M. I., Singh, H. et al. (2007). Evaluating drug prices, availability, affordability, and price components: implications for access to drugs in Malaysia. *PLoS Medicine*, 4(3).

Barber, S. L., Huang, B., Santoso, B. et al. (2013). The reform of the essential medicines system in China: a comprehensive approach to universal coverage. *Journal of Global Health*, 3(1).

Bennett, S., Quick, J. D., Velásquez, G. et al. (1997). Public-private roles in the pharmaceutical sector-implications for equitable access and rational drug use.WHO/DAP/97.12. Geneva: World Health Organization.

Brudon, P. , Rainhorn, J. D. & Reich, M. R. (1994). Indicators for monitoring national drug policies: a practical manual. *World Health Organization Action Programme on Essential Drugs C.*

Cameron, A. (2010). Cost savings of switching consumption from originator brand medicines to generic equivalents. World health report 2010. < http://www. who. int/healthsystems/topics/financing/healthreport/whr _ background/en>

Cameron, A., Ewen, M., Ross-Degnan, D. et al. (2009). Medicine prices, availability, and affordability in 36 developing and middle-income countries: a secondary analysis. *Lancet*, 373(9659).

CFDA. (2012). Implementation plan about the pilot work on designated production. <http://www.sda.gov.cn/WS01/CL0844/76196.html>

Charles, W. F. & Lu, X. Q. (2011). *Implementing health care reform policies in China*. Washington, D.C. : Center for Strategic and International Studies.

Chaudhury, R. R., Parameswar, R., Gupta, U. et al. (2005). Quality medicines for the poor: experience of the Delhi programme on rational use of drugs. *Health Policy Plan*, 20(2).

Chen, D. W., Shen, T. B., Hu, L. et al. (2012). Compensation mechanism of basic medical institutions after implementation of essential drug system in Zhejiang Province. *Joural of Chinese Rural Health Service Administration*, 32(8).

Chen, W., Tang, S., Sun, J. et al. (2010). Availability and use of essential medicines in China: manufacturing, supply, and prescribing in Shandong and Gansu Provinces. *BMC Health Serv Res*, 10.

China NDRC. (2009a). Implementation plan for the recent priorities of the health care system reform (2009-2011). <http://www.sdpc.gov.cn/shfz/yywstzgg/ygzc/t20090408_359821.htm>

China NDRC. (2009b). Opinions of the CPC Central Committee and the State Council on deepening the Health Care System Reform. <http://www.sdpc.gov.cn/shfz/yywstzgg/ygzc/t20090408_359822.htm>

China NDRC. (2011). Government report on the centralized procurement of essential medicines. < http://www.sdpc.gov.cn/shfz/yywstzgg/ygdt/t20111122_445785.htm>

Chinese Ministry of Health. (2009). National essential medicines List for primary health institutions. <http://www.gov.cn/gzdt/2009-08/18/content_1395524.htm>

Chinese MoH. (2011a). China health statistical yearbook (2011).

Chinese MoH. (2011b). Implementation progress of national essential medicine system. <http://www.moh.gov.cn/mohywzc/s7652/201110/53137.shtml>

Dye, T. R. (2010). *Understanding public policy* (13 edn.). New York: Pearson Education, Inc.

Lu, C.Y., Ross-Degnan, D., Stephens, P. et al. (2013). Changes in use of antidiabetic medications following price regulations in China (1999-2009). *Journal of Pharmaceutical Health Services Research*, 4.

Currie, J., Lin, W.C., Zhang, W. (2010). Patient Knowledge and Antibiotic Abuse Evidence from An Audit Study in China. *NBER Working Paper Series Working Paper 16602*. Cambridge: National Bureau of

Economic Research.

Deepak, P. (2006). Rational use of drugs: the challenging need for developing countries. *CARE Nepal Newsletter*, 9(1).

Desalegn, A. A. (2013). Assessment of drug use pattern using WHO prescribing indicators at Hawassa University teaching and referral hospital, south Ethiopia: a cross-sectional study. *BMC Health Serv Res*, 13, 170.

Diaz, R., Behr, J. G. & Tulpule, M. (2012). A system dynamics model for simulating ambulatory health care demands. *Simul Healthc*, 7(4).

Dong, L. F., Wang, D. L, Gao, J. H. et al. (2011). Doctor's injection prescribing and its correlates in village health clinics across 10 provinces of western China. *J Public Health*, 33(4).

Dubnick, M. J. & Bardes, B. A. (1983). *Thinking about public policy*. New York: Wiley.

Eggleston, K., Li, L., Meng, Q. Y. et al. (2008). Health service delivery in China: a literature review. *Health Econ*, 17(2).

Euro Health Group & MSH-Tanzania. (2007). United Republic of Tanzania Drug Tracking Study Report. United Republic of Tanzania.

Goh, Y. M. & Love, P. E. D. (2012). Methodological application of system dynamics for evaluating traffic safety policy. *Safety Science*, 50.

Guan, X. & Shi, L. (2009). Research on China Essential Medicine System. *Journal of China Pharmaceutical*, 44(2).

HAI. (2008). Global andregional core list. <http://www.haiweb.org/medicineprices/updatesMay2008/GlobalRegCoreMedsMay08.pdf>

Halfdan, M. (2009). *Thirty years of essential medicines: the challenge*. Valencia: Farmamundi.

Helen Y. (2013). Essential medicines reform in China. <http://www.wpro.who.int/china/topics/essential_medicines/faq/en/index.html>

Hill, S., Henry, D. & Stevens, A. (2001). The use of evidence in drug selection:the Australian pharmaceutical benefits scheme. In D. M. Fox & A. D. Oxman (eds.), *Informing judgement: case studies of health policy and research in six countries* (pp. 7-28). New York: Milbank Memorial Fund.

Hou, J. L., Li, N., Lu, L. et al. (2011). Research on Shanghai resident satisfaction of primary healthcare after new health reform. *Chin J Hosp Admin*, 27(10).

Hu, S. L., Zhang, Y. B. & Ye, L. (2007). Research on national basic medicine system. *Health Economics Research*, (10).

Huang, T. T., Dong, Y. Q., Wang, X. X. et al. (2011). Analysis of the rural outpatients' cognition on essential medicines policy and their medicine behaviors. *Journal of Chinese Rural Health Service Administration*, 32(4).

Thamrin-Akib, H.R. (2005). Indonesia: poster competition spreads the rational use message. *Essential drugs monitor*, 34.

Iizuka, T. (2007). Experts' agency problems: evidence from the prescription drug market in Japan. *Rand J Econ*, 38(3).

Isah, A., Ross-Degnan, D., Quick, J. et al. (1997). The development of standard values for the WHO drug use prescribing indicators. <http://www.icium.org/icium1997/posters/1a2_txt.html>

McDavid, J.C. & Hawthorn, L. R. L. (2006). *Program evaluation and performance measurement: an introduction to practice*. California: Sage Publications, Inc.

Jiang, Q., Yu, B. N., Ying, G.Y. et al. (2012). Outpatient prescription practices in rural township health centers in Sichuan Province, China. *BMC Health Serv Res*, 12.

Kar, S. S., Pradhan, H. S. & Mohanta, G. P. (2010). Concept of essential medicines and rational use in public health. *Indian J Community Med*, 35(1).

Kotwani, A., Ewen, M., Dey, D. et al. (2007). Prices & availability of common medicines at six sites in India using a standard methodology. *Indian J Med Res*, 125(5).

Kumar, S. (2011). Modeling patient flow operation of a US urban county hospital. *Technol Health Care*, 19(4).

Hayford, K., Privor-dumm, L. & Levine, O. (2011). Improving access to essential medicines through public-private partnerships. International Vaccine Access Center.

Lester, J. P. & Stewart, J. (2000). *Public policy* (2 edn.). Belmont, CA: Wadsworth Publishing Company, Inc.

Li, X. (2009). *Social system dynamic policy reasearch: theory, method and its application*. Shanghai: Fudan University Press.

Li, X. T., Wang, W. H. & Yin, A. T. (2011). Study on the impact of essential medicine system on rational drug use in township hospitals of Shandong Province. *Chinese Health Economics*, 30(4).

Li, Y., Ying, C., Sufang, G. et al. (2013). Evaluation, in three provinces, of the introduction and impact of China's National Essential Medicines Scheme. *Bull World Health Organ*, 91(3).

Liu, P. (2013). How to solve the difficult problem of essential medicines' supply: based on the public governance theory. *Chinese Journal of Health Policy*, 6(3).

Lofgren, H. & Boer, R. (2004). Pharmaceuticals in Australia: developments in regulation and governance. *Soc Sci Med*, 58(12).

Mamdani, M. (1992). Early initiatives in Essential Drugs Policy. In N. Kanjiet al. (eds.), *Drugs Policy in Developing Countries*. London: Zed Books.

Mankiw, N. G. (2007). *Macroeconomics*. New York: World Publishers.

Hoarda, M., Homerb, J. & Manley, W. (2005). Systems modeling in support of evidence-based disaster planning for rural areas. *International journal of hygiene and environmental health*, 208.

Maynard, A. & Bloor, K. (2003). Dilemmas in regulation of the market for pharmaceuticals. *Health Affairs*, 22.

Mhamba, R. & Mbirigenda, S. (2010). The drugs industry and access to essential medicines in Tanzania *EQUINET Discussion Paper Series* 83. Harare: Training and Research Support Centre, SEATINI, Rhodes University, EQUINET.

MOHRSS. (2009). Per capita annual net income of rural households by sources and region. <http://www.mohrss.gov.cn/2010/html/0183.htm>

Morgan, S., McMahon, M. & Greyson, D. (2008). Balancing health and industrial policy objectives in the pharmaceutical sector: lessons from Australia. *Health Policy*, 87(2).

MSH. (2009). International drug price indicator guide. <http://erc.msh. org/mainpage.cfm? file=1.0.htm&module=DMP&language=english>

Mui, F. G. & Chee, W. G. (2012). China's pharmaceutical distribution: poised for change. <http://www. atkearney. com/paper/-/asset_publisher/ dVxv4Hz2h8bS/content/china-s-pharmaceutical-distribution-poised-for-change/ 10192#sthash.UkrzTXnR.dpuf>

National Bureau of Statistics of China. (2010). National statistical database for consumer price index. < http://219. 235. 129. 58/reportView. do? Url =/ xmlFiles/01e3c6636bee425ab325dbf869d601d8. xml&id=520d35a792644d97be7a84 ab1ecb8c15&bgqDm=20100000&i18nLang=zh_CN>

Norman, R. (2001). National drug policy: implications of the tough on drugs' ideology. *Collegian: Journal of the Royal College of Nursing Australia*, 8(4).

OECD. (2005). Drug spending in OECD countries up by nearly a third since 1998, according to new OECD data. <http://www.oecd.org/document/ 25/0,2340,en_2649_37407_34967193_1_1_1_37407,00.html>

Pavin, M., Nurgozhin, T., Hafner, G. et al. (2003). Prescribing practices of rural primary health care physicians in Uzbekistan. *Tropical Medicine and International Health*, 8(2).

Pei, S. (2011). Interview on China's essential medicine system. Retrieved May 18, 2012. < http://news. 163. com/11/1114/19/7IRGKTTM00014JB5. html>

Pinto C. P. B. S., Miranda, E. S., Emmerick, I. C. M. et al. (2010). Medicine prices and availability in the Brazilian Popular Pharmacy Program. *Rev Saude Publica*, 44(4).

Quick, J. D. (2003). Essential medicines twenty-five years on: closing the access gap. *Health Policy Plan*, 18.

Quick, J.D., Hogerzeil, HV, Velasquez, G. et al. (2002). Twenty-five years of essentials medicines. *Bulletin World Health Organization*, 80(11).

Senarathna, S. M. D. K. G., Mannapperuma, U., Fernandopulle, B. M. R. (2011). Medicine prices, availability and affordability in Sri Lanka. *Indian J Pharmacol*, 43(1).

Shao, R. Q., Zuo, G. Y. & Zhao, L. (2009).Discussion on Construction of National Essential Drug policy under the Circumstances of New Health Reform. *Chinese Pharmaceutical Affairs*, 23(2).

Song, Y. & Bian, Y. (2011a). Discussion on the social cost of public hospital reform based on drug addition income from 2003 to 2009. *Journal of Chinese Pharmaceutical Affairs*, 25(12).

Song, Y. & Bian, Y. (2011b). Impact analysis of "Zero-profit" policy on drug price reduction in primary health institutions. *China Pharmacy*, 22(44).

Song, Y. & Bian, Y. (2011c). Impact evaluation of essential medicine system in primary health care institutions of Zhejiang Province. *Chinese Journal of Health Policy*, 4(10).

Song, Y. & Bian, Y. (2012a). Empirical study of China's essential medicine system on improving access to medicines. *Chinese Journal of Health Policy*, 5(7).

Song, Y. & Bian, Y. (2012b). Impact evaluation of essential medicine system on prescription charges in township hospitals of Shandong province. *Journal of Chinese Health Service Management*, 8.

Song, Y. & Bian, Y. (2012c). Impact of the essential drug list on rational drug use in grassroots facilities. *Journal of Health Economics Research*, 9.

Song, Y. & Bian, Y. (2013a). Analysis on changes of drug price after implementing of the essential drug system in primary health care institutions-based on the empirical study of the four provinces (autonomous regions) in China. *Chinese Journal of Health Economics Research*, 4.

Song, Y. & Bian, Y. (2013b). Cognition and satisfaction survey of primary health workers on national essential medicine system in Ningxia rural areas. *Chinese Rural Health Service Administration*, 33(2).

Song, Y. & Bian, Y. (2013c). Investigation and survey of effects of national Essential Drug System on township hospitals in Shandong Province and its policy suggestions. *China Pharmacy*, 21(8).

Soumerai S. (1998). Factors influencing prescribing. *American Journal of Health Promotion*, 18.

Sterman, J. (2000). *Business dynamics—system thinking and modeling for a complex world*. Boston: McGraw-Hill Higher Education.

Sun, J. (2009). How to formulate and implement national medicines policy: experiences and lessons learnt from India for China. *Chinese Journal of Health Policy*, 2(6).

Sun, Q., Santoro, M. A., Meng, Q. et al. (2008). Pharmaceutical policy in China. *Health Aff (Millwood)*, 27(4).

Tian, X., Song, Y. & Zhang, X. (2012). National essential medicines list and policy practice: a case study of China's health care reform. *BMC Health Serv Res*, 12.

Wang, D. & Zhang, X. (2011). The selection of national essential medicines in China: progress and the way forward. *Southern Med Review*, 4(1).

Wang, L., Yu, J. J., Zhou, B. M. et al. (2009). A systematic review of national drug policy in seventeen countries. *Chin J Evid-based Med*, 9(7).

Wang, Q. & Chen, W. (2010). Analysis on essential medicines policy with new institutional economics. *Chinese Journal of Health Policy*, 3(6).

Wang, X. L., Zheng, Z. Q., Qu, S. M. et al. (2011). Short-term effectiveness of zero-profit essential drugs policy evaluated by the stakeholders of grassroots medical institutes. *Journal of Chinese General Practice*, 14(4A).

Wang, Y. P., Liu, J. W., Chen, J. et al. (2011). Analysis of present compensation mode of essential medicine system in China. *Joural of China Pharmacy*, 22(8).

Weersuriya, K. & Brudon, P. (1998). Essential drugs concept needs better implementation.*Essential Drugs Monitor*, 25 & 26.

WHO. (1987). The rational use of drugs: report.

WHO. (1993a). A short information manual on the Tanzania National Drug Policy. < http://collections. infocollections. org/whocountry/en/d/ Jh4335e/2.1.html>

WHO. (1993b). How to investigate drug use in health facilities: selected drug use indicators.

WHO. (1995). Contribution to updating the WHO guidelines for developing national drug policies.

WHO. (2000). WHO medicines strategy: framework for action in essential drugs and medicines policy 2000-2003.

WHO. (2001a). Updating and disseminating the WHO model list of essential drugs: the way forward. <http://dcc2.bumc.bu.edu/richardl/WHO _Select_docs/whoedlprocess15May31_eng.doc>

WHO. (2001b). Global strategy for containment of antimicrobial resistance. WHO Communicable Disease Surveillance and Response (CSR).

WHO. (2002a). Report on the 12th Expert Committee on the selection and use of essential medicines.

WHO. (2002b). The selection of essential medicines. WHO policy perspective on medicines.

WHO. (2002c). Promoting rational use of medicines: core components.

WHO policy perspectives on medicines.

WHO. (2003a). Access to essential medicines: a global necessity. Essential Drugs Monitor No. 032.

WHO. (2003b). Essential drugs and medicines policy: supporting countries to close the access gap.

WHO. (2003c). How to develop and implement a national drug policy.

WHO. (2004a). Model formulary.

WHO. (2004b). WHO medicine strategy (2004-2007): countries at the core.

WHO. (2004c). The world medicines situation. rational use of medicines. <http://apps.who.int/medicinedocs/en/d/Js6160e/10.html>

WHO. (2007a). Better medicines for children. <http://www.who.int/childmedicines/publications/WHA6020.pdf>

WHO. (2007b). Operational package for assessing, monitoring and evaluating country pharmaceutical situations: guide for coordinators and data collectors.

WHO. (2009). Country pharmaceutical situations.

WHO. (2011a). Comparative table of medicines on the WHO Model List of Essential Medicines from 1977-2011. < http://www.who.int/entity/medicines/publications/essentialmedicines/EMLsChanges1977_2011.xls>

WHO. (2011b). Median availability of selected generic medicines. <http://www.who.int/gho/mdg/medicines/situation_trends_availability/en/index.html>

WHO. (2011c). WHO model lists of essential medicines. <http://www.who.int/medicines/publications/essentialmedicines/en/index.html>

WHO. (2012a). The pursuit of responsible use of medicines: sharing and learning from country experiences.

WHO. (2012b). WHO/Health action international project on medicine prices and availability. <http://www.who.int/medicines/areas/access/Medicine_Prices_and_Availability/en/index.html>

WHO. (2013a). Essential medicines. < http://www.who.int/topics/essential_medicines/en/>

WHO. (2013b). Essential medicines and pharmaceutical policies. <http://www.emro.who.int/entity/essential-medicines/>

WHO. (2013c). Essential medicines list: 30 years of vital health care. < http://www.allcountries.org/health/essential_medicines_list_eml.html>

WHO. (2013d). WHO model lists of essential medicines. <http://www. who.int/medicines/publications/essentialmedicines/en/index.html>

WHO/HAI. (2003). Medicine prices: a new approach to measurement.

WHO/HAI. (2008). Measuring medicine prices, availability, affordability and price components.

World Bank. (2010a). Financing, pricing, and utilization of pharmaceuticals in China: the road to reform.

World Bank. (2010b). PPP conversion factor, private consumption (LCU per international $). <http://search. worldbank .org/data? qterm = Purchasing+Power+Parity>

Xiao, Y., Zhao, K., Bishai, D. M., et al. Essential drugs policy in three rural counties in China: what does a complexity lens add? *Social Science & Medicine*, 93.

Xinhuanet. (2010). Drug prices decreased by about 30%. <http://news. xinhuanet.com/politics/2010-12/24/c_12914270.htm>

Xu, J., Fang, G. X. & Jiang, Q. C. (2011). Analyzing the prescription cost in village clinics of rural Anhui. *The Chinese Health Service Management*, 1.

Yan, K. K., Yang, S. M., Fang, Y., et al. (2010). KAP survey of the cognition of 377 primary doctors on national essential drug system. *Joural of China Pharmacy*, 21(44).

Yang, H. Y., Sun, Q., Zuo, G. Y., et al. (2012). Changes of drugs' usage and structure of township hospitals under Essential Medicine System: cases in three counties of Shandong Province. *Chinese Health Economics*, 31 (4).

Yang, L., Liu, C., Ferrier, J. A. et al. (2013). The impact of the National Essential Medicines Policy on prescribing behaviours in primary care facilities in Hubei Province of China. *Health Policy & Plan*, 28(7).

Yang, L., Luo, M., Jin, C. H. et al. (2012). Comparative study on essential drug centralized bidding purchase plans of provinces in China. *Joural of China Pharmacy*, 23(16).

Ye, L. (2009). *A study of national essential medicines system*.

Shanghai: Fudan University Press.

Ye, L., Hu, S. L., Ewen, M.et al. (2008). Evidence-based study on the affordability of essential drugs in Shanghai. *Journal of Chinese Health Resources*, 11(4).

Yoongthong, W., Hu, S. L., Whitty, J. A. et al. (2012). National drug policies to local formulary decisions in Thailand, China, and Australia: drug listing changes and opportunities. *Value in Health*, 15(1).

Yu, X., Li, C., Shi, Y. et al. (2010). Pharmaceutical supply chain in China: current issues and implications for health system reform. *Health Policy*, 97(1).

Yuan, Q. & Tang, S. L. (2012). Comparative analysis of compensation model of essential drug system and its compensation mechanism research. *Journal of China Medical Herald*, 9(30).

Zhang, Q. Y., Yin, Y. Q., Wei, J. et al. (2011). Satisfaction on the pilot project of National Essential Drug System in doctors at township hospitals of Chenzhou, Hunan Province. *Chinese Journal of Practical Preventive Medicine*, 18(8).

Zhang Y.B., Hu, S. L., He, J. J. et al. (2010). Preliminary analysis of pharmaceuticals zero mark-up policy in Shanghai. *Chinese Journal of Health Policy*, 3(6).

Zhu, H. (2004). Research on the demand elasticity of drugs in China. *China Pharmacy*, 15(11).

Zhu, J. J., Wang, W. J. & Jiang, Q. C. (2012). Analysis on operation status of primary healthcare facilities before and after medicine zero-profit policy. *Chinese Journal of Soft Science of Health*, 26(7).

Zhuo, J., Sleigh, A. C. & Wang, H. (2002). Unsafe injection and HIV transmission in Guangxi, China. *Chinese Medical Journal*, 115(6).

Appendices

Appendix I：Questionnaire of hospital general information

表2：基层医疗卫生机构基本情况抽样调查表

所在省：_____   所在市：_____

机构名称：_____

单位负责人：_____

机构类型：□中心乡镇卫生院   □一般乡镇卫生院   □社区卫生服务中心

国家基本药物制度实施时间：   年   月[1]

指标名称	计量单位	2008年	2009年	2010年	2011年[2]
一、基本情况					
1. 门急诊人次数	人次				
2. 门诊处方数	张				
3. 出院人数	人次				
二、收支情况					
4. 总收入	元				
其中：门诊收入	元				
内：门诊药品收入	元				
住院收入	元				
内：住院药品收入	元				
5. 　财政补助收入（含上级补助）	元				
6. 总支出	元				
7. 　其中：药品支出	元				
三、基本药物使用情况					
8. 本机构配备的药物品种数	种				
9. 　其中：国家基本药物品种数[3]	种	/			
10. 　省级增补药物品种数	种	/			
11. 药品销售总额	元				
12. 　其中：国家基本药物销售额	元	/			
13. 　　省级增补药物销售额	元	/			
14. 本机构全年申购药品金额数	元				
15. 　其中：按合同要求及时配送金额	元				
16. 本机构全年申购药品次数	次				
17. 　其中：及时配送次数	次				

填表人：_____   联系电话（手机）：_____

填报日期：   年   月   日

填表说明：

[1]实施基本药物制度判断标准：实现了省级招标、统一配送，政府办基层医疗卫生机构全部配备使用基本药物并实现零差率销售；

[2]统计数据时间截止到2011年6月底；

[3]按照《国家基本药物目录》说明中方法统计目录内药物品种数。

Appendix II: Questionnaire of medicine prices

表3：基本药物价格变化情况调查表，含表3(a)、表3(b)

填表说明：

1. 填写本医疗机构内所有配备使用的国家基本药物目录和省级增补药物目录中的药品，条目不够请自行增加。其中，表3(a)为国家基本药物目录内药品情况，表3(b)为省补基本药物目录内药品情况；

2. 只填写2009年6月1日至30日，2010年6月1日至30日和2011年6月1日至30日同时在使用的，且剂型和规格相同的药品；

3. 零售价和月销售金额以元为单位，只填写数字，不填写单位；

4. 填表示例：

项目	目录范围	序号	基本药物名称（通用名）	剂型	规格	2009年6月		2010年6月		2011年6月	
						零售价（元）	月销售金额（元）	零售价（元）	月销售金额（元）	零售价（元）	月销售金额（元）
目录类型	国家基本药物目录中的药品	1	头孢呋辛酯片	片剂	250mgX12片/盒	52.49	1574.7	40.1	1443.6	38.5	1540
		2	注射用头孢呋辛钠	注射剂	750mg/支	37.19	743.8	28.26	621.72	28.2	846
		3									
		4									

表3(a)：国家基本药物目录内药品价格变化情况调查表

填报机构：　　　　　　　　　　　　　　　　　　　　　　　　　　填报日期：　　年　　月　　日

项目	目录范围	序号	基本药物名称（通用名）	剂型	规格	2009年6月		2010年6月		2011年6月	
						零售价（元）	月销售金额（元）	零售价（元）	月销售金额（元）	零售价（元）	月销售金额（元）
目录类型	国家基本药物目录中的药品	1									
		2									
		3									
		4									
		5									
		6									
		7									
		8									
		9									
		10									
		11									
		12									
		13									
		14									
		15									
		16									
		17									
		18									
		19									
		20									
		21									
		22									
		23									
		24									
		25									
		26									
		27									
		28									
		29									
		30									

填表人：　　　　　　　联系电话（手机）：

Appendix III: Questionnaire of satisfaction
on NEMS for rural residents

医院患者对基本药物制度的
满意程度调查

您好！首先非常感谢您能参与我们此次问卷调查。本问卷就旨在了解公众对基本药物制度的满意程度，以评价现阶段各基层医疗机构基本药物制度的执行效果，更好地促进国家基本药物制度的完善、保证基本药物的可及和合理使用。答案无所谓对错，请您按照自己的体会与看法填写。我们大约会占用您 10 分钟的时间。本次问卷调查不记姓名，调查结果仅用于学术研究，我们保证会对您所提供的所有信息予以严格保密。

再次衷心感谢您的支持与合作！

澳门大学基本药物制度课题组

2011.12

A 个人基本情况

（以下问题在有横线处填写具体内容，在有方框"□"处有选择性地打钩）

A1. 看病的科室：_____科

A2. 性别：□ 男_____ □ 女

A3. 出生日期：_____年_____月

A4. 文化程度：□ 大学及以上　□ 大专　□ 高中/中专　□ 初中　□ 小学及以下

A5. 家庭总收入平均每月为：

□ 1000 元以内　□ 1000~1999 元　□ 2000~2999 元　□ 3000~4999 元

□ 5000 元以上

A6. 付费类别：

□ 新农合　□ 城镇职工医疗保险　□ 城镇居民医疗保险　□ 自费

□ 其他（请注明_____）

B 对基本药物制度的认知

（以下问题在有横线处填写具体内容，在方框"□"处有选择性地打钩）

B1. 您知道国家基本药物制度吗？

□ 非常熟悉　　□ 熟悉　　□ 了解一点　　□ 听说过　　□ 不知道

B2. 您知道基本药物在乡镇卫生院实行零差率销售吗？

□ 非常熟悉　　□ 熟悉　　□ 了解一点　　□ 听说过　　□ 不知道

B3. 您知道基本药物的相关报销政策吗？

□ 非常熟悉　　□ 熟悉　　□ 了解一点　　□ 听说过　　□ 不知道（跳过 B4）

B4. 您对基本药物的报销政策满意吗？

□ 很满意　　　□ 比较满意　　□ 一般　　　□ 不满意　　　□ 很不满意

C 对基本药物价格的感知（以下问题在方框"□"处有选择性地打钩）

C1. 您觉得基本药物制度实施之后在乡镇卫生院看病的总花费有下降吗？

□ 大大下降了　　□ 略有下降　　□ 没变化　　□ 略有增加　　□ 大大增加了

C2. 您觉得基本药物制度实施之后乡镇卫生院的药品价格有下降吗？

□ 大大下降了　　□ 略有下降　　□ 没变化　　□ 略有增加　　□ 大大增加了

C3. 现阶段您对乡镇卫生院的总体收费满意吗？

□ 很满意　　□ 比较满意　　□ 一般　　□ 不满意　　□ 很不满意

C4. 现阶段您对乡镇卫生院药品的价格满意吗？

□ 很满意　　□ 比较满意　　□ 一般　　□ 不满意　　□ 很不满意

D 对基本药物质量和品种的感知（以下问题在方框"□"处有选择性地打钩）

D1. 现阶段您对乡镇卫生院基本药物的质量满意吗？

□ 很满意　　　□ 比较满意　　□ 一般　　　□ 不满意　　　□ 很不满意

D2. 您认为基本药物的疗效与其他药物相比有什么不同吗？

□ 更好很多　　□ 稍好一些　　□ 相同　　□ 较差一些　　□ 差很多

D3. 您对"乡镇卫生院只配备和使用基本药物"认同吗？

□ 很认同　　　□ 比较认同　　□ 不太认同　　□ 很不认同　　　□ 无所谓

D4. 医院现有的基本药物品种能满足您的药品需求吗？

□ 满足且过于富余　　□ 满足且略有富余　　□ 恰好满足　　□ 略不够用

□ 完全不够用

E 对医院药事服务态度的感知（以下问题在方框"□"处有选择性地打钩）

E1. 卫生院里医务人员的服务态度和以前相比有变化吗？

□ 变好了很多　　□ 稍有改观　　□ 没变化　　□ 略不如以前　　□ 比以前差很多

E2. 现阶段您对卫生院药师的服务态度满意吗？

□ 很满意　　　□ 比较满意　　□ 一般　　□ 不满意　　□ 很不满意

E3. 现阶段您对医院药师给予用药指导的程度满意吗？

□ 很满意　　　□ 比较满意　　□ 一般　　□ 不满意　　□ 很不满意

F 您对基本药物制度总体满意吗？

（0～10 分，请给出您的评分，并在分数对应的"□"内打钩）

非常不满意————————————————→非常满意

□　　□　　□　　□　　□　　□　　□　　□　　□　　□　　□

0　　1　　2　　3　　4　　5　　6　　7　　8　　9　　10

G 您认为医院还应该多配备哪些品种的基本药物？（请填写）_____

调研员（签字）：_____

日　期：_____年____月____日

Appendix Ⅳ: Questionnaire of satisfaction on NEMS for primary health workers

医务人员对基本药物制度的
满意程度调查

您好！首先非常感谢您能在百忙之中参与和协助我们完成此次问卷调查。本问卷旨在了解公众对于基本药物制度的满意程度，以评价现阶段基层医疗机构基本药物制度的实施效果，更好地促进国家基本药物制度的完善，保证基本药物的可及和合理使用。答案无所谓对错，请您按照自己的体会与观点填写。我们大约会占用您 10 分钟的时间。本次问卷调查不记姓名，调查结果仅用于学术研究，决不涉及商业用途和个人隐私，我们保证将对您所提供的所有信息予以严格保密。

再次衷心感谢您的支持与合作！

澳门大学基本药物制度课题组
2011.12

A 个人基本情况

（以下问题在有横线处填写具体内容，在有方框"□"处有选择性地打钩）

A1. 性别:□ 男　　□ 女

A2. 出生日期:_____年____月

A3. 工作年限:_____年

A4. 文化程度:□ 大学及以上　□ 大专　□ 高中/中专　□ 初中　□ 小学及以下

A5. 所在科室/专业:
□ 内科　□ 外科　□ 妇产科　□ 儿科　□ 眼科　□ 皮肤科　□ 耳鼻喉科
□ 急诊　□ 药房　□ 护理　　其他(请注明_____)

A6. 职称等级:□ 士级　　□ 初级　　□ 中级　　□ 高级

A7. 月均收入:
□ 1000 元以内　　□ 1000～1999 元　　□ 2000～2999 元
□ 3000～4999 元　　□ 5000 元以上

B 对基本药物制度的认知

（以下问题在有横线处填写具体内容，在有方框"□"处有选择性地打钩）

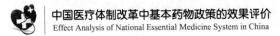

B1. 您了解国家基本药物制度吗

☐ 非常熟悉　　☐ 熟悉　　☐ 了解一点　　☐ 听说过　　☐ 不知道

B2. 您了解国家基本药物目录吗？

☐ 非常熟悉　　☐ 熟悉　　☐ 了解一点　　☐ 听说过　　☐ 不知道

B3. 您接受过基本药物制度的相关培训吗？

☐ 接受过（请注明＿＿＿＿＿＿次）　　　　☐ 没有接受过

C 对基本药物制度的感知（以下问题在方框"☐"处有选择性地打钩）

C1. 您对基本药物的定价满意吗？

☐ 很满意　　　☐ 比较满意　　　☐ 一般　　　☐ 不满意　　　☐ 很不满意

C2. 您对基本药物的质量满意吗？

☐ 很满意　　　☐ 比较满意　　　☐ 一般　　　☐ 不满意　　　☐ 很不满意

C3. 您认为基本药物的疗效与其他药物相比有什么不同？

☐ 更好很多　　☐ 稍好一些　　☐ 相同　　☐ 较差一些　　　☐ 差很多

C4. 您认为现有基本药物能满足临床常见疾病的诊治需求吗？

☐ 满足且过于富余　　☐ 满足且略有富余　　☐ 恰好满足　　☐ 略不够用　　☐ 完全不够用

C5. 您认为基本药物实行零差率销售会减少患者的药物经济负担吗？

☐ 会大幅减少　　☐ 会稍微减少　　☐ 不产生影响　　☐ 会小幅增加　　☐ 会大幅增加

C6. 实施基本药物零差率销售后，您所在科室的收入是否受到影响？

☐ 大大增加了　　☐ 略有增加　　☐ 没变化　　☐ 有所减少　　☐ 大大减少了

C7. 实行基本药物制度后，您的工资水平是否受影响？

☐ 大大增加了　　☐ 略有增加　　☐ 没变化　　☐ 有所减少　　☐ 大大减少了

C8. 您赞同大力普及基本药物制度吗？

☐ 很赞同　　　☐ 比较赞同　　　☐ 不太赞同　　　☐ 很不赞同　　　☐ 无所谓

D 您对基本药物制度总体满意吗？

（0～10 分，请给出您的评分，并在分数对应的"☐"处内打钩）

非常不满意————————————————→ 非常满意

☐	☐	☐	☐	☐	☐	☐	☐	☐	☐	☐
0	1	2	3	4	5	6	7	8	9	10

E 您认为医院还应该多配备哪些品种的基本药物？（请填写）＿＿＿＿＿＿＿＿＿＿＿＿＿

调研员（签字）：＿＿＿＿＿＿＿＿

日期：＿＿＿＿年＿＿＿月＿＿＿日

Appendix V: Interview outline

基层医疗卫生机构基本药物制度
实施情况访谈提纲

（供访问人员用）

访问人员：澳门大学基本药物制度课题组

访问对象：市（县）卫生局、医改办、药监局、各乡镇卫生院/社区卫生服务中心的负责人等

访谈题目：基层医疗卫生机构基本药物制度实施情况

访谈目的：了解基层卫生医疗机构基本药物政策的执行情况；掌握基本药物制度实施过程中存在的主要问题和各方对未来的改革期望；了解基本药物制度与其他制度及改革措施的衔接情况；了解基本药物制度实施前后对医疗卫生服务带来的影响。

您好！很高兴能有这样一个机会向各位请教，首先非常感谢诸位能抽出宝贵的时间参与我们的研究。

我们是澳门大学国家基本药物制度课题组的成员。为了能进一步了解基层医疗卫生机构基本药物制度的实施情况，掌握基本药物制度实施过程中存在的主要问题和各方对未来的改革期望，我们特别组织了此次访谈。对于各位的支持和配合，我们表示十分感谢。

整个访谈过程约1～2小时。在访谈中，我们将会按照您手中的访谈提纲向您请教一些问题，访谈内容包括：

1）您所在市（县）的基本药物制度相关政策介绍；

2）基本药物制度实施前后，您所在市（县）医疗机构医疗卫生服务的变化情况；

3)您在基本药物制度实施过程(包括采购、配送、定价和使用等)中遇到的问题、所采取的应对策略以及对未来改革方向的建议;

4)基本药物制度与其他医改举措的衔接问题。

1. 基本药物制度的实施对基层医疗卫生机构产生了哪些影响?回答内容至少应包括:

1)门诊和住院患者的数量有无变化?减少或增加?百分比是多少?

2)配备药品品种数有没有变化?减少或增加?百分比是多少?

3)药品的价格和销售数量有无变化?减少或增加?百分比是多少?

4)医院收入有无变化?减少或增加?百分比是多少?

5)医务人员的待遇有无变化?

2. 现有基本药物目录的品种能否满足基本医疗卫生机构就诊患者的需求?哪些品种尚需补充?

3. 对于基层医疗机构只能配备和使用基本药物,您怎么看?这样是否会限制有条件的基层卫生院的诊疗范围?特别对于一些慢性病患者、简单的外科手术等,该如何去用药、处理?

4. 各地目前已经在 307 种国家基本药物的基础上增扩了目录,宁夏相对于其他省份增补品种较少(仅 64 种),宁夏在制定省级增补目录时主要考虑了哪些补充因素?

5. 基本药物的报销比例是否高于非基本药物报销比例?高出多少?

6. 基本药物制度之后,财政补偿是否充足、到位?您认为应该在目前的形势下对基层医疗机构采取什么样的补偿政策较适合?

7. 医疗机构基本药物的进货渠道、采购模式,以及采购的频次、遴选标准是什么?

8. 药品"三统一"实施的情况如何?遇到的主要问题是什么?

9. 中标药品的配送情况如何?是否出现部分基本药物配送短缺问题?配送覆盖率大约为多少?

10. 基本药物的招标及其他医疗保险药品目录的招标有无重复设置?这两个制度是如何衔接的?

11. 卫生院和辖区内卫生室的药品供应存在什么关系?是否已实施乡村一体化?

12. 医院药品使用规范的执行和培训情况怎么样?有无开展?

13. 您认为现阶段卫生院需要解决的最重要的问题是什么?为什么?

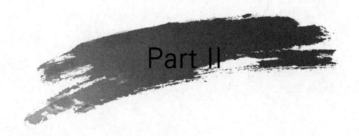

Part II

List of Abbreviations

ADR	Adverse Drug Reaction
API	Active Pharmaceutical Ingredient
CBA	Cost-benefit Analysis
CEA	Cost-effectiveness Analysis
CFDA/CDR	Center for Drug Reevaluation of China Food and Drug Administration
CHC	Community Health Center
CH	County-level Hospital
CMB	China Medical Board
CUA	Cost-utility Analysis
DDD	Defined Daily Dose
DRG	Diagnosis-related Group
DSPRUD	Delhi Society for the Promotion of Rational Use of Drugs
EBM	Evidence-based Medicine
EFA	Exploratory Factor Analysis
EM	Essential Medicine
EML	Essential Medicine List
GDP	Gross Domestic Product
INRUD	International Network for the Rational Use of Drugs
IRP	International Reference Price
MLR	Multiple Linear Regression
MoH	Ministry of Health

MSH	Management Science for Health
NDRC	National Development and Reform Commission
NEMS	National Essential Medicine System
NF	National Formulary
NHCR	New Health Care Reform
NHFPC	National Health and Family Planning Commission
NMP	National Medicine Policy
NSAID	Nonsteroidal Anti-inflammatory Drug
PBS	Pharmaceutical Benefits Schedule
PCA	Principal Component Analysis
PEML	Provincial Supplementary Essential Medicine List
PHC	Primary Health Care
PHI	Primary Health Institution
RUM	Rational Use of Medicines
SDUI	Selected Drug Use Indicator
SLR	Simple Linear Regression
SREB	Separation of Revenue and Expenditure Budgets
STG	Standard Treatment Guide
TCM	Traditional Chinese Medicine
THC	Township Health Center
UNICEF	United Nations International Children's Emergency Fund
VHC	Village Health Clinic
WHA	World Health Assembly
WHO	World Health Organization
WHO/DAP	WHO's Action Programme on Essential Drugs
WM	Western Medicine
WPRO	WHO Regional Office for the Western Pacific

Chapter 1　Introduction

1. 1　Background

1. 1. 1　Issue of rational medicine use

With the swift development of economy since the 1980s, medical and health services in China have got considerable improvement. The most internationally-recognized three essential indicators for describing the health of a population could reflect this great progress. Life expectancy increased to 74. 8 in 2010 from 67. 9 in 1981 (China Public Health and Family Planning Statistical Yearbook, 2015a), infant mortality rate dropped to 8. 9‰ in 2014 from 34. 7‰ in 1981 by 74% (China Public Health and Family Planning Statistical Yearbook, 2015a; China Public Health and Family Planning Statistical Yearbook, 2015b), maternal mortality rate dropped to 21. 7 per 100,000 in 2014 from 80. 0 per 100,000 in 1991 by 73% (China Public Health and Family Planning Statistical Yearbook, 2015b). Many of advanced medical technologies and treatments that meet the constantly growing need of the population for curing and preventing diseases have been introduced, which also promote the development of the pharmaceutical industry, medicine logistics, hospital etc. in China.

However, behind this brilliant progress, widespread use of medicines leads to very high costs which creates enormous economic burden on the population, exacerbates the disparity of health service across the regions with different socio-economic status, and lowers the efficiency of health resources use. (Wang, Lin & Dong, 2000) Health expenditure per capita rose to 2581. 7 *yuan in* 2014, more than 200 times than that in 1978 (see Figure 1-1). (China Public Health and Family Planning Statistical Yearbook, 2015c) In the year of 2014, average medicine expense per outpatient and per inpatient of hospitals was 106. 3 *yuan* and 2999. 8 *yuan*, accounting for 48. 3% and 38. 3% of outpatient and inpatient cost, respectively, while in primary health institutions, the number for community health centers (CHCs) was 63. 5 *yuan* and 1162. 1 *yuan*, accounting for 68. 8% and 44. 1%, respectively, and the number for township health centers (THCs) was 30. 9 CNY and 633. 4 CNY, accounting for 54. 3% and 45. 8%, respectively. (China NHFPC, 2014) Figure 1-2 describes the changes of average medicine expense per outpatient and per inpatient in hospitals, CHCs and THCs from 2001 to 2014. The average medicine expense per patient went up rapidly during this period with a little fluctuation. Even more serious was the fact that inappropriate or the irrational use of medicines could be liable to serious adverse drug event (ADR), which might cause physical impairment, deformity, disability or even death.

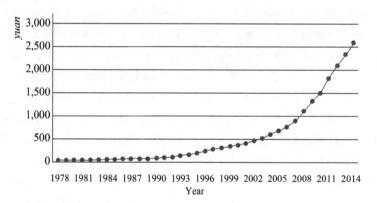

Figure 1-1   Health expenditure per capita in China (1978-2014)

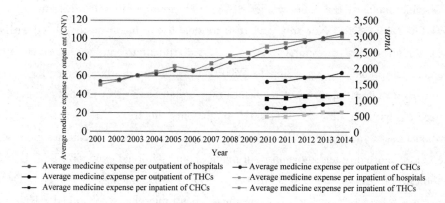

Figure 1-2　Medicine expense per patient in China (2001-2014)[1]

The rational use of medicines or the rational use of drugs was first proposed by the World Health Organization in Nairobi, 1985, following the initiation of study on medicine application in 1970s. "Patients receive medications appropriate to their clinical needs, in doses that meet their own individual requirements, for an adequate period of time, and at the lowest cost to them and their community." (WHO, 1985) However, RUM is not a static normative paradigm, but a dynamic process of management and decision-making involving medical sciences, social science and market force. From a medical angle, medicine application is influenced by physicians' proficiency in diagnosis and familiarity of medicines. From a social point of view, medicine use is restricted by differences in values, social relationships and psychosocial elements between physicians and patients. And from economic aspect, price and affordability of medicines, as well as coverage and payment of medical insurance play important roles in medicine approach. For these complicated subjective and objective reasons, the prevalence of the irrational use of medicines and its grave consequences has become a global public health issue, drawing much attention of regulators, communities and researchers in health field.

There are various forms of the irrational use of medicines, for instance, excessive use of medicines, abuse of antibiotics and injections, making a prescription

---

① Source: Statistical bulletin of the health development in China, 2001-2014.

disobeying standard treatment guides (STGs), inappropriate self-medication, etc. (WHO, 2003a; 2006) Not only does the irrational use of medicines is related with a large amount of health resources, but also it is detrimental to individual patient and the general population. According to WHO, 14% of the deaths around the world result from the irrational use of medicines rather than diseases or natural aging, and instead of dying of illness itself, 33% of patients die from ADR caused by the irrational use of medicines. (WHO, 2002d) The irrational use of medicines increases the risk of morbidity and mortality, bringing about additional expenditure of £ 470 million every year in the UK. (Hitchen, 2006; Pirmohamed et al., 2004). Drug resistance that was generated by the abuse of antimicrobials consumed additional health resources of $ 4-5 billion in US and € 9 billion in Europe in 2005 respectively. (Levy, 2005; Verhoef et al., 2005) Overuse of injections has increased the risk of bloodborn diseases, such as hepatitis B and C, AIDS etc. (Simonsen et al., 1999)

Retrospective study investigating the prescriptions in health institutions is one of the standard methods for medicine utilization research recommended by WHO, as prescription analysis provides robust evidence for understanding existing circumstance of medicine use and prescribing behaviors of health workers, as well as to improve rational medicine use (WHO, 1993). This study method has been widely applied in developing and transitional countries. According to WHO, one third of deaths were attributed to irrational use of medicines, more than half of medicines were inappropriately prescribed, distributed or sold around the world, and more or less 50% of patients were not capable of taking medicines on time and in dose complying with physicians' instructions. (WHO, 2002d; 2009b) Ample research evidences illustrate that medicine use is not on the way to rationality. (WHO, 2006) In developing countries, the percentage of encounters with an antibiotic prescribed was 40%-50%, much higher than the recommended scale of 20.0%-26.8%, and the average number of medicines per encounter increased from 2 to 2.5, also exceeding the reference standard of 1.6-1.8. (WHO, 2011b) In developed countries, the irrational use of medicines was also a problem that was not completely settled. Even in the Netherlands, a country with less usage of antibiotics, National Health Services Survey indicated that antibiotics were misused to treat 6 diseases that did not necessarily need antibiotic therapy. For instance, 6% of children with asthma and 67.2% of patients with nasosinusitis adopted antibiotic treatment .

In China, most of medicine utilization studies are conducted after the year of 2000. (Tu, 2013) The studies find that the antibiotic utilization for outpatients was more than 50%, and the usage of intravenous drip and hormone was over 30% and 8% respectively. The Center for Drug Reevaluation of China Food and Drug Administration (CFDA/CDR) investigated medicine treatment for children in 26 hospitals from Beijing, Wuhan, Chongqing, Guangzhou, etc. in 2004, finding that the rational use of medicines for diarrhea accounted for only 5.4%, and merely 12.3% of the medicine treatments for pneumonia were appropriate. (Tian & Yu, 2005) Abuse of antibiotics was the most common and severe incorrect medicine use in China. 90% of upper respiratory infection (URI) and 70% of diarrhea were not recommended to be treated fed by using antibiotics, but health workers tended to prescribe them when treating these two diseases. More than 60% of patients with URI adopted antibiotic treatment (Jin & Zhou, 2009), and in some health institutions, the number even reached to 90%. (Lv, Guo, Zhong & Yan, 2009). Only 40.5%-45.8% of inpatients with infantile diarrhea were detected as infectious diarrhea, but 99% of them took antibiotics. (Huang & Zhou, 2011; Ke, 2008). The irrational use of medicines has become a serious public health issue in China, urging the government to take steps.

1.1.2 New healthcare reform and essential medicine policy of China

China launched its new healthcare reform (NHCR) program in April 2009, which aimed to settle a series of problems that existed in the health system. One of the five core components of the program is that efforts should be made to establish the National Essential Medicines System (NEMS) in order to secure pharmaceutical supply and ensure medicine safety. A major mission of NEMS is to improve rational medicine therapy, and the policy is globally implemented in developing countries. (WHO, 1987; 1988; 1993) The medicines selected for the Essential Medicines List (EML) are carefully evaluated and screened to ensure their necessity, safety, effectiveness and cheapness, and should be used with high priority and rationally in health institutions throughout the country in accordance with the policy requirement. The availability of EML is one cornerstone for rational prescribing, based on which the implementation of formulary and medicine use guideline that is tailored to the local medical needs and physicians' skills could bring about improvements in the availability and rational use of medicines.

China's NEMS, along with the other four key matters of the NHCR, which include the basic medical insurance, improvement of primary healthcare delivery system, equalization of basic public health service, and public hospital reform, establish a complex system encompassing seven interrelated parts, namely medicine selection, production, pricing, procurement, delivery, utilization and reimbursement. The newly built NEMS, in light of the concept expressed by WHO, aims to improve medicine availability, affordability and rational use, as well as to cut the profit link between health facilities, doctors and medicines. The NEMS of China was implemented in primary health institutions (PHIs) initially, and PHIs were required to outfit essential medicines (EMs) only. (Song, 2013)

The relation between RUM and NEMS will be described in detail in Chapter 2.

1.1.3　Primary health care and RUM in rural areas of China

80% of the 1.3 billion Chinese population live in rural areas. That every rural resident can have access to primary health care (PHC) is one of the major objectives of the rural health service in China. The Outline for Development of Rural Primary Health Care in China (2001-2010) proposes to improve the rural health service system, to perfect the service functions, to implement diversified rural medical security systems, to settle the problems of basic healthcare and prevention for rural residents, and to boost the rural residents' health and life quality by deepening the reform. (China MoH, 2002)

Accordingly, Ministry of Health (MoH, now renamed as National Health and Family Planning Commission, NHFPC), along with United Nations International Children's Emergency Fund (UNICEF), launched a promotion program for rural PHC in 2001, in order to enhance the diagnosis and treatment for common and frequent diseases in rural three-tier health service network: county level, township level and village level. (Nie, Yao, Lu & Chen, 2002) This program fully investigates the irrational use of medicines and its impact factors in the village healthcare clinics (VHCs) from selected rural areas, and takes adequate actions, with favorable effects of reduction of antibiotics and hormones use, frequency of injection administration, average number of medicines used in a prescription, as well as prescription charges. (Nie et al., 2002; Yao et al., 2002). Nevertheless, the investigation on the irrational use of medicines in township health centers. (THCs), which are the most essential PHIs for rural PHC, is not intensive and thorough enough. (Fu, Sun, Sun, & Lu, 2004) Likewise, for county-level hospitals (CHs) which provide rural PHC with major technical support, there is deficiency of quantitative information and evaluation on RUM. (Yao et al., 2002) Therefore, it is necessary to assure the situation of irrational medicine use and its impact factors in county and township level health institutions so as to make an overall evaluation on RUM in rural PHC and thus to present counter measures and strategies.

1. 1. 4 Existing study on medicine utilization in China

Most researches on prescriptions to investigate RUM in China are following the guidance manual named "How to investigate drug use in medical facilities: Selected drug use indicators" (SDUIs) contributed by WHO's Action Programme on Essential Drugs (WHO/DAP) and the International Network for the Rational Use of Drugs (INRUD) in 1993. (Tu, 2013) Not only does the SDUIs contain medicine utilization information, but also it involves humanity concern over physicians' and pharmacists' service, so as to evaluate the medicine therapy status scientifically and impartially in a health institution. (Chen, 2011) The SDUIs consist of 12 core indicators, which are divided into three groups: prescribing indicators, patient care indicators and health facility indicators, and another seven complementary indicators. (WHO, 1993) Prescribing indicators have been widely applied among the studies on medicine utilization in China, while other indicators, in particular patient care indicators are almost absent from the existing researches. Meanwhile, there is no comprehensive evaluation method to integrate the indicators so as to give an overall judgment of RUM in a health institution.

The SDUIs method essentially requires random sampling on a large number of prescriptions to ensure representativeness, but few of the existing literatures in China have adequately explain this, making the results less reliable. WHO report indicates that, it is a limitation of the report that the available data are insufficient in this enormous market of medicine consumption with a large population. (WHO, 2004)

In addition, a few studies to analyzing the factors that affect RUM, and some referring to the influences on RUM are generally about physicians' prescription behavior and its motivation instead of health institutions' organizational barriers associated with the achievement of RUM.

1. 2　Research objectives

RUM in the vast rural areas concerns the health of three quarters of the Chinese population, and is an essential public issue of rural PHC which the NHCR pledged an endeavor to improve. Researches on medicine utilization there are helpful for approaching medicines safely, effectively and economically for rural residents. By investigating the prescriptions from rural three-tier health institutions, this study aims to estimate RUM for outpatients in rural areas of China under the context of NHCR, and to establish a comprehensive evaluation method for RUM tentatively. Besides, organizational barriers associated with the achievement of RUM are also identified, according to which policy recommendations and strategies are proposed.

1. 3　Potential contributions

Firstly, evaluation of RUM under the context of the NHCR will discover the effects of the policies, especially the NEMS, to some extent. It could provide information and recommendations for the further reform and play an indispensable role in policy improvement.

Secondly, this study investigates the existing circumstances of RUM by the SDUIs using samples from the rural areas of seven provinces in western China, so that the results of this study are comparable as a baseline among areas and over time. The detailed methods can be easily replicable, and the results produced from big raw data are representative.

Thirdly, there is no existing method to integrate the SDUIs and to give a comparable overall score to judge RUM in a health institution, and this study makes an effort to establish a synthetic appraisal index. Therefore, the verdict on RUM can be used for further deep-going researches.

Last but not least, identifying the organizational barriers associated with the achievement of RUM is conducive to promote the management of public health institutions, as well as to optimize some supporting policies and strategies, such as financial subsidies.

1. 4　Design and organization

As is shown in Figure 1-3, to achieve the objectives, this study will review the literatures to illustrate the concepts and relevant policies, as well as to summarize the fundamental state of RUM in health institutions and the research progress both at home and abroad. Then, statistical analysis will be conducted by processing the data from field study, including descriptive statistics, univariate and multivariate analysis, principal component analysis (PCA) etc., with IBM SPSS 19. 0 software. Evaluation will be made according to theoretical analysis and data results. Policy implications will be also proposed to deal with the practical issues, based on this research.

Seven interrelated chapters are included in Part II as below:

Chapter 1 describes the background of this research, which corresponds to the detriment that results from the irrational medicine use, types of the irrational use of medicine and current situation of RUM. Meanwhile, the relevant public health subjects and system reform are introduced. Also, existing related works are briefly summarized. In addition, the whole picture, including research objectives, potential contributions, conceptual framework of this research etc., is presented in this chapter.

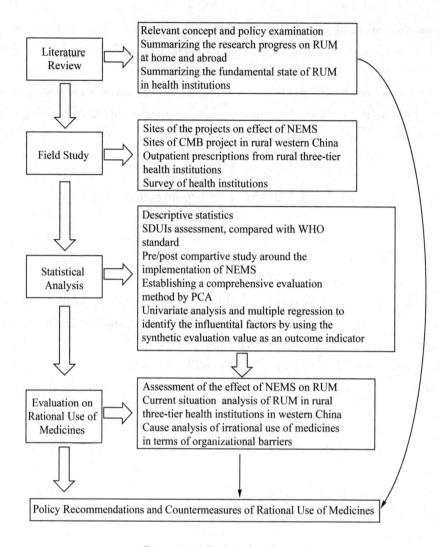

Figure 1-3　Technical pathway

Chapter 2 generalizes and summarizes the related theories by literature review, in order to set up a theoretical foundation and clarify the logical connection between RUM and related public health subjects and policies, inclusive of NEMS, along with the existing strategies to promote RUM. The SDUIs method to evaluate RUM is also overviewed, on the basis of which the comprehensive evaluation method will be established.

Chapter 3 explains the research methodology in detail, and specifies the implementation approach of this research, including data sampling and collection，data processing and analysis and data quality assurance.

Chapter 4 presents the effect of the NEMS on RUM，based on investigations carried out in THCs from four provinces with different socio-economic status in China by using the pre/post comparative study. It provides very early baseline data on RUM after the NHCR was introduced.

Chapter 5 presents the current situation of RUM in rural three-tier health institutions sampling from seven provinces in western China. Furthermore，by conducting PCA with these data，a comprehensive evaluation method is tentatively established，generating a synthetic assessment value for further study.

Chapter 6 presents the results of analysis of influences in terms of organizational factors of health institutions，using the synthetic assessment value as an outcome indicator of RUM. Organizational barriers associated with the achievement of RUM is identified，providing a basis of health institutions management improvement.

Chapter 7 is the conclusion and it provides some policy recommendations and strategies based on the results. Also，the limitations of this research are illustrated and the prospective works are previewed.

Chapter 2　Literature Review

2.1　The concept of RUM

2.1.1　WHO definition of RUM

WHO arranged a meeting named "Conference of Experts on the Rational Use of Drugs", in Nairobi, Kenya, during 25-29 November, 1985. The meeting discussed ways of ensuring RUM, in particular through improved knowledge and flow of information, and the role of marketing practices in this respect, especially in developing countries, concerning governments, pharmaceutical industries, and patients' and consumers' organizations. It was stated in the meeting that RUM required the medications that patients receive should be appropriate to their clinical needs, in order to meet their own individual requirements, and at the lowest cost to the patients and the community. It was for the first time that RUM was explicitly defined, after the initiation of study on medicine application in the 1970s.

WHO put forward the criterion of RUM in 1987 as follows:

(1) Prescribed drugs should be appropriate medications;

(2) Ensuring the supply of medications at affordable prices to the public, at the appropriate time;

(3) Dispensing correctly;

(4) Taking medications in precise dosage, right usage and proper duration;

(5) Ensuring the safety and effectiveness of medications.

In 1997, the implication of RUM was amended by WHO and Management Sciences for Health (MSH) as: to use medicines safely, effectively and economically. (WHO/DAP, 1997) The specific requirements included:

(1) Correct medicines;

(2) Appropriate indication;

(3) Appropriate efficacy, safety, suitability and affordability to the patients;

(4) Appropriate dosage, administration and duration;

(5) No contraindication to patients, foreseeable ADR at a minimum;

(6) Correct dispensing, including proper medicine information for patients;

(7) Good patient adherence to treatment.

2.1.2　The principles of RUM

The later definition of RUM mentioned above emphasizes the correspondence of indications and medications as well as patient care. Yet, the four principles of RUM are constant: safety, effectiveness, economy and appropriateness. (Suleman, 1997)

Medicine utilization is risky, but in order to cure diseases and relieve pains, people have to take a certain risk. Therefore, safe medication is the foundation of RUM. It is not the principle that effect should be the best; instead, to pursue a point at which the treatment effect is optimal while the risk is relatively low makes more sense. This treatment principle is concrete, on the basis of specific individuals and medications. The safety of a medicine is a relative concept with limiting conditions, which means that it will not usually bring about harms to the patients with appropriate indications of the medicine in appropriate dose. However, as human body is a complicated system, there are great disparities from person to person, so that ADR may be generated to somebody with particular constitution from a medicine that is safe for the majority of people. For the patients whose life are endangered by some medical condition, it is necessary to use the medications that has the best effect and serious ADR, but adequate measures to reduce the side effects should be also taken.

中国医疗体制改革中基本药物政策的效果评价
Effect Analysis of National Essential Medicine System in China

Effectiveness of medicine means the treatment effect must be definite. For instance, antihypertensives should necessarily reduce patients' blood pressure to a certain extent, and asthma drugs are bound to relieve the symptom of patients' dyspnea promptly. Effectiveness is the primary goal of medication and the general performance of interaction between medicines and human bodies. Due to the distinctions among medicine users in terms of age, constitution, severity of illness etc., the treatment effect is not identical. Most people will receive a feedback after taking the medicine.

Economy does not simply mean whether medicine price or treatment charge is high or not, but it refers to an interrelationship between medicine cost and therapeutic effectiveness or benefit. Economy of RUM does not simply seek an expense cut, nor purport to use medicines in line with the principle of the cheaper, the better or the less, the better. Economy is aimed at the advance of the efficiency of medication resources in less cost and more effect, deriving cost-effectiveness analysis (CEA), cost-utility analysis (CUA) and cost-benefit analysis (CBA).

Appropriateness is the fundamental assurance to achieve RUM, embodied in all aspects of medicine use. It refers to right medicine selection, appropriate dosage, proper administration route, adequate combined medication etc., in order to make medicines into full play, reduce ADR, restrain the development of diseases and recuperate people's health.

These four principles are integral, only with which RUM could be achieved. (Jiang, Wang & Jin, 2005)

2.1.3 The concept of RUM is not constant

With the development of medical sciences, new treatments have been emerging endlessly, and old therapies are being gradually replaced. Many medications once supposed to be the best have been eliminated, so RUM is basically not an absolute concept but a relative idea in accordance with the evolution of medical sciences and social-economic conditions.

· 170 ·

2. 2　The specifications of RUM

2. 2. 1　Choosing medications based on the characteristics of disease is the premise of RUM

2. 2. 1. 1　Based on the pathogenesis and clinical manifestation

Clinicians have to fully realize the characteristics of disease on the basis of definite diagnosis, understanding pathogenesis, clinical manifestation, disease course and potential development, so as to select medications with favorable curative effect, low side effect and high pertinency. The pharmacology of chosen medications should be sufficiently understood as well, including indications, contraindications, dosage, administration route, timing of administration, and basis of combined use.

2. 2. 1. 2　Based on the severity and type of disease

A medical condition is likely to involve primary disease and complications with different severity and urgency, so the medication protocol has to place priority on the more principal ones, making a trade-off according to the subjective and objective conditions as well as advantages and disadvantages to patients.

2. 2. 1. 3　Based on the effect evaluation

The medication protocol has to be adjusted if there is no remarkable effect, searching for causes and changing medicines and the ways of use by medical history collection, complete inspection and diagnosis examination.

2. 2. 2　Approaching medicines based on their characteristics

2. 2. 2. 1　Medicine properties

The physical and chemical properties of medicine determine its function. For example, nanoparticle-delivered medicine is being wide applied nowadays, with better effect and lower side effect as well as in no higher dose than needed due to the active agent deposited only in the morbid region.

2. 2. 2. 2　Dosage

Different dosage results in different effect. Generally, within certain limit, the higher concentration of medicine in blood is, the stronger effect medicine produces. However, excessive dosage may lead to toxic reactions. For instance, escalating dosage of atropine is likely to experience palpitation, mydriasis, flushing, dysphoria and mental disorder successively.

2. 2. 2. 3　Dosage form and administration route

Each medicine produces optimal effect by providing the dosage form and the administration route is appropriate. And different preparations of same active pharmaceutical ingredient (API) can produce different degrees of effect. Generally speaking, injection takes effect much more significantly than oral medicine since its uptake is faster. Solution is easier to be absorbed than tablet and capsule among oral medicines. In addition, some medicines take various effects via different administrations. For example, magnesium sulfate has an effect of catharsis by oral intake, while by intramuscular injection or intravenous drip it takes effect of sedation and intracranial pressure reduction.

2. 2. 2. 4　Combination of medications

In order to achieve the goal of treatment, sometimes it is necessary to adopt two or more medicines simultaneously or successively. By combination medications can interact with one another in vivo or in vitro, thus affecting medicine efficacy and safety. There is a variety of medicines available nowadays, and combination of medications is widely adopted, so ADR caused by the interaction of medicines should concern the crowd.

2. 2. 2. 5　Long-term medication

Some diseases require long-term medication, so tolerance, dependency and withdrawal reaction of medicine have to be watched.

2. 2. 3　Personalized medication based on individuals' organic trait

2. 2. 3. 1　Hereditary factor

Genetic polymorphism can affect the effect of medicine on human body in terms of effector organs, histocytes, metabolic enzymes, receptors and so on.

2. 2. 3. 2　Physiological factor

Age, weight, gender etc. should be taken into account in medication. For instance, children's tissues and organs are in growth and development, so improper use of medicines can induce dysgenopathy and more serious ADR, an leave sequela. Women in the condition of gestation or lactation should be cautious of medication.

2. 2. 3. 3   Pathological factor

Many morbid conditions can affect medicine effect by means of changing medicine characteristics of pharmacokinetics and pharmacodynamics as well as pharmacological interaction. In clinical practice, for patients who have not only got the principal disease, but also tend to suffer from other medical conditions, dosage or administration route of medication has to be adjusted to avoid serious side effect or futile treatment, especially for hepatic, nephritic or cardiac conditions.

2. 2. 3. 4   Psychological factor

Psychological activity can have an influence on medication efficacy, usually in chronic, functional and mild diseases.

2. 2. 3. 5   Life style and environment

Diet, nutriture as well as living and working environment may affect medicine action.

2. 2. 3. 6   Time rhythm

Medicine effect can be influenced by changes of biological rhythm as well, in terms of time-medicine effect, chronic toxicity and time-medicine metabolism.

2. 2. 3. 7   Individual variation

Some individuals are susceptible to medication, and tend to take lower dose intake than normal, while some other individuals have to adopt medication at higher dose before it takes effect. (Chen, 2011)

2. 3   Summary of irrational use of medicines

2. 3. 1   Patterns of irrational use of medicines

Common patterns of irrational prescribing of medicines can be manifested in the following forms:

(1) The use of medicines, when no medication is indicated;

(2) The use of an incorrect medicine for a specific condition requiring medication;

(3) The use of medicines with dubious or unproven efficacy;

(4) The use of medicines of uncertain safety status;

(5) Failure to provide available, safe and effective medicines;

(6) The use of correct medicines with incorrect administration, dosage and duration;

(7) The use of unnecessary expensive medicines.

Some instances of commonly encountered, inappropriate prescribing practices in many health care context include:

(1) Overuse of antibiotics;

(2) Indiscriminate use of injections;

(3) Abuse of hormones;

(4) Polypharmacy.

2.3.2 Situation of irrational use of medicines

Since the 1950s, there has been an upsurge of the research and development of new medicines in developed countries. Thousands of medicines have been approved, and combinations of medications and long-term medications are on the increase. (Zhao & Miao, 2001) While the increase of medicines that provide more options in clinical treatment, the irrational use of medicines and ADR increase constantly. Drug-induced diseases and antibiotic resistance become more and more severe around the world, causing heavy burdens on individuals and the community. (Asscher, Parr & Whitmarsh, 1995) A survey on misuse of medicines in 1,081 hospitals of US in 1992 with a sample size of 430,000 indicates that 5.22% of inpatients in US received incorrect medicines every year; that is to say, there was one medication error in every 19.13 inpatients on average, and there were 90,895 victims of medication error every year. (Bond, Raehl & Franke, 2002) It is estimated that permanent disability and death caused by medication error led to a loss of $76.6 billion in health institutions of US in 1995, of which 20% was hospitalization expense and 18% was long-term medication cost. (Johnson & Bootman, 1995). The expenditure for drug-induced reactions had exceeded the cost of medicines itself in US. (Manasee, 1989) A study shows that unnecessary and irrational self-medications with antibiotics were common in Europe as well.

In developing countries, the situation of irrational use of medicines was even worse due to backward medical technology and health management. A survey on prescriptions in India reveals medicine exposure to the patients, as well as indiscriminate use of nonsteroidal anti-inflammatory drug (NSAIDs), antibiotics and vitamins increased. (Rishi, Sangeeta, Surendra & Tailang, 2003) An analysis of 9,678 prescriptions in Afghanistan shows that over 50% of all outpatients were prescribed at least one antibiotic, and most of the antibiotic-prescribed prescriptions were without a recorded diagnosis. (Bajis et al., 2014) Odusanya says in a paper that in Lagos, Nigeria, the injections were prescribed for a variety of indications where oral therapy could have been used, and antibiotics were prescribed largely for presumed infections. (Odusanya, 2004) A study about western Nepal points out that only 13% of medicines were prescribed by generic name, the percentage of medicines prescribed from EML of WHO or home was less than 50%, rate of antibiotics encountered was 28.3%, and average cost per prescription was about $3.73. (Ghimire et al, 2009) A study in Sudan finds that rates for improper prescribing and dispensing practices and prevalence of self-medication with antibiotics were staggering high, and indicators of rational medicine use had deteriorated over the past decade in spite of the implementation of managerial, regulatory and training interventions. (Awad, Ball & Eltayeb, 2007) Medicine utilization in a Brazilian pediatric hospital between September 2012 and February 2013, indicates that the prevalence of off-label and unlicensed utilization of medicines were 20.9% and 77.8% respectively, and polypharmacy was highly associated to both off-label and unlicensed regimen.

WHO believed that irrational use of medicines was an urgent and widespread problem in both public and private health sectors in both developed and developing countries. A lot of countries did not have a stringent authority for medicine regulation nor an integrated national program or body to promote RUM. There were insufficient attention and resources towards prescribers, dispensers and consumers for coping with the problem of irrational use of medicines.(WHO, 2007a)

In China, Tang Jingbo, panel leader of CFDA/CDR, estimates that irrational use of medicines accounted for 12%-32% of all medications, and around 190,000 inpatients died of ADR every year. (Tang & Li, 2011) In 2009, medicine charges for outpatients and inpatients accounted for 50.7%

and 44.0% of total medical expenses respectively (China MoH, 2009), while in developed countries the proportions were 10%-30% (Kleinke, 2001). Abuse of antibiotics and hormones, as well as indiscriminate use of injections has become the most prominent problem of irrational use of medicines in China. An investigation indicates that every inpatient in Chinese hospitals received more than 2.5 bottles/bags of infusion daily on average, with each bottle/bag containing 2 vials of intravenous injections. (Wu & Jiao, 2010) Millions of people in China caught a common cold every year, and more than 80% of them received unnecessary injections of antibiotics. While 50% of people who encountered a medical condition adopted antibiotics, only 25% of the adoptions were necessary. Half children who have got a symptom of cough or running nose would be treated with antibiotics by their parents. In consequence, 60%-70% of bacteria developed medicine resistance through these abuse of antibiotics. (Sun, 2010; Tang & Li, 2011) Glucocorticoids were widely applied in China to abate a fever or elevate blood pressure for the critical patients with influenza, pulmonitis, shock, etc. but without infectious shock or adrenaline fall, leading to rise of virus titer and prolongation of virus elimination, hence exacerbation of the disease. (Tang & Li, 2011; WHO, 2009a). There are diversified manifestations of irrational use of medicines in China, e.g. medication without a clear indication, medicine incompatibility, violation of medicine contraindication and caution, excessive or insufficient dosage, over-length or too-short duration, inadequate dosage form and administration, as well as overmuch polypharmacy. (Su, Su & Yang, 2008; Zhou & Yang, 2009) A study on outpatient prescriptions in a tertiary hospital shows that among irrational use of medicines, incorrect administration and dosage accounted for 17.11%, repeated medication accounted for 16.93%, inappropriate combination of medicines accounted for 13.45%, non-correspondence between medication and diagnosis accounted for 9.61%, pharmacologic antagonism accounted for 8.78%, incompatibility of medicines accounted for 8.60%, improper medicine selection accounted for 7.50%, incorrect medicine dosage form and specifications accounted for 6.95%, excess of medicines (more than 5 medicines in one prescription) accounted for 5.76%, and dissolvent mismatch accounted for 5.31%. (Wang, 2009)

2. 3. 3　Consequences of irrational use of medicines

Irrational use of medicines creates serious consequences for patients, the public, the health system, and even the economy, in terms of poor patient outcome, ADR, increasing antibiotics resistance, and wasting resources.

2. 3. 3. 1　Delayed treatment

Medication with incorrect indication, under-dose, too-short duration, pharmacologic antagonism etc. can reduce medication efficacy, and results in delayed treatment, aggravation of disease and treatment failure. (Aronson, 2004)

2. 3. 3. 2　ADR and drug-induced diseases

A large proportion of medicines have some certain toxicity that is detrimental a to human body. Medication is a trade-off. Incorrect use of medicines can generate ADR and drug-induced diseases. (Aronson, 2004)

2. 3. 3. 3　Medication accident

Serious and irreversible injury brought about by inappropriate medicine use with personal responsibility can be a medication accident. (Zhu et al., 2009)

2. 3. 3. 4　Waste of health resources

Medicine resources even health resources would be wasted by irrational use of medicines. Tangible waste is manifest as firsthand over-consumption, while intangible waste, which is usually neglected by health workers and patients, is caused by increasing unnecessary consumption to tackle ADR and drug-induced diseases. (Qu, 2004)

2. 3. 4　Influences on irrational use of medicines

There are various factors that affect the irrational use of medicines like those deriving from patients, pharmacies, prescribers, the workplace, the supply system, industry influences, regulation, drug information and misinformation. (Khan & Ara, 2011)

Physicians have been assigned a gatekeeper role for health care (Willems, 2001), and as prescribers they are gatekeepers of RUM. Inappropriate prescribing is a manifestation of irrational medicine use. (MSH, 2012) Prescribing is a complex task requiring diagnostic skills, knowledge of medicines, an understanding of the principles of clinical pharmacology, communication skills, appreciation of risk and uncertainty. (Troup, 1989) In fact, physicians prescribe in diversified circumstances, often in the absence of evidence. Rational prescribing decisions normally follows a logical sequence from diagnosis to follow-up, and must be based on knowledge interpreted according to many other factors. (Khan & Ara, 2011) On the basis of the characteristics of the medical work, limited by the macroscopic social environment, the health system and hospital rules, prescribing behavior is a habit manifested from prescribers' medical knowledge and clinical experiences. In addition, in many places, prescribers may include paramedics, nurses and drug sellers who have received relatively less training in the use of medicines, so their irrational prescribing practices have to be considered as well.

Nevertheless, adequate knowledge on rational medicine use does not always result in rational prescribing behavior. (Hogerzeil, 1995) Market mechanism is likely to fail in health sector due to the specificity of health service, for instance, polypharmacy and excessive use of expensive medicines leading to a waste of resources. (Cheng, 2003) Among the participants: drug maker and distributor, hospital and physician, and patient, hospital and physician play a core role in the medicine market. On one aspect, medical providers monopolize the asymmetric information; on the other aspect, they are healthcare proxies, so they can achieve the market superiority and manipulate the volume and the price. (Chen, Sun & Zhao, 2006) Prescribers make decisions on what, how many and how medicines should be used in clinical medication, so it is essential to monitor, normalize and guide prescribers' prescribing behavior in order to promote RUM in health institutions.

Table 2-1 summarizes the principal factors that can influence irrational use of medicines.

Table 2-1   The principal factors that influence irrational use of medicines

Factors	Main manifestations
Human Factors	
Physician Factor	Insufficient knowledge on ingredients, pharmacokinetics, ADR, interaction etc. of medicine

Continued

Factors	Main manifestations
Pharmacist Factor	Poor prescription review, poor medication guide, poor medication monitoring etc.
Nurse Factor	Inadequate medicine feed, absence of monitoring
Patient Factor	Non-adherence
Medicine Factors	
Medicine Nature	Efficacy and ADR
Medicines Interaction	Combined use results in interactions among medicines; The more medicines, the higher possibility
Medicine Quality	Poor medicine quality reduces efficacy and increasing occurrence of ADR
Socio-environmental Factors	
Medicine Pricing Policy	New medicines and brand-name medicines produce numerous profit; old medicines and generic medicines are of low price and slim margins
Hospital Compensatory Mechanism	"Drug-maintaining-medicine" makes medical providers tend to prescribe more expensive medicines, in larger quantity, in order to achieve higher benefit
Medication supervision	Poor ADR monitoring and reporting, poor pharmacovigilance, lack of adequate laws and regulations
Social and Cultural Psychology	Patient incorrect knowledge and habit on medication, or conflicting cultures and conventions

2.4   Interventions to promote RUM

2.4.1   WHO core strategies

WHO advocated 12 key interventions to promote more RUM in 2002:

(1) Establishment of a multidisciplinary national body to coordinate

policies on medicine use;

(2) Use of clinical guidelines;

(3) Development and use of national EML;

(4) Establishment of drug and therapeutics committees in districts and hospitals;

(5) Inclusion of problem-based pharmacotherapy training in undergraduate curricula;

(6) Continuing in-service medical education as a licensure requirement;

(7) Supervision, audit and feedback

(8) Use of independent information on medicines

(9) Public education about medicines

(10) Avoidance of perverse financial incentives

(11) Use of appropriate and enforced regulation

(12) Sufficient government expenditure to ensure availability of medicines and staff.

Most of the strategies are mutually supportive. Monitoring medicine use and using the collected information to develop, implement and evaluate strategies to change inappropriate medicine use behavior are fundamental to any national program to promote RUM. A mandated multi-disciplinary national body to coordinate all actions and sufficient government funding are critical to success. (WHO, 2002d)

2.4.2 Characterizing interventions

Interventions to improve RUM can be characterized as either targeted directly towards prescribers, e.g. education, managerial or administrative tactics, or system-oriented, which focus on policies, regulations and economic strategies.

In educational interventions, prescribers are persuaded by information or knowledge provided in the form of face-to-face education or training, seminars, and provision of written materials. Follow-up and monitoring are necessary to make the interventions more effective and sustainable. In addition, patients are provided with consultation and information through face-to-face medication directions and public media.

In managerial interventions, prescribers are guided in the decision-making process, by limiting lists for routine procurements, medicine use review and feedback, supervision and monitoring, provision of National Formulary (NF) and STGs, and monitoring of prescribers' use of the formularies and guidelines.

In regulatory interventions, prescribers are squeezed to restrict decision-making process in prescribing. These strategies incorporate policies stimulating use of generic medicines, limitations on prescribing and dispensing, and recall of questionable medicines in the market.

In economic interventions, prescribers are motivated by the promotion of positive financial incentives and the avoidance of vicious incentives. The economic strategies include changes in reimbursement for health providers, e.g. public or private insurance plan, capitation-based reimbursement, and quality-based performance. Moreover, setting aside medicine sales by prescribers removes the financial incentive for excessive prescribing.

Interventions can also be characterized as preventive or curative. Preventive approaches ensure the prescribers behave in an appropriate way. Curative interventions try to reverse a pattern of irrational use of medicines. Prevention is much easier and more effective than curing, which is always true in medications. (MSH, 2012)

2.4.3 Intervention effect

Many interventions have a certain effect in a certain setting. Over time, interventions have to follow up prescribers' behaviors and are improved in time; regions, health care organizations, local communication channels, level of education, and other factors affecting the effectiveness of specific strategies in different contexts have to be taken into account, in order to make interventions succeed when transferring from one setting to another. (MSH, 2012)

Figure 2-1 displays intervention outcomes found in various studies in 2009. 108 studies are included, and in each line, mark means median impact of largest change in medicine use outcome discovered in the studies, and terminal vertexes represent the upper and lower quartiles respectively.

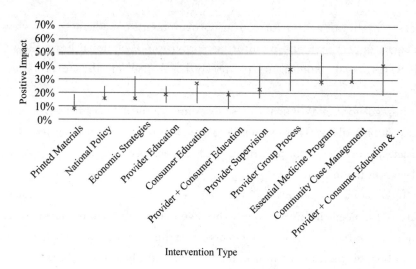

Figure 2-1   Intervention impact outcomes (2009)①

2.4.4   Interventions on RUM in China

Along with initiation of the NHCR, a systematic NEMS was established in 2009. New national EML reduced the number of medicines outfitted in PHIs and narrowed the options of medicines for prescribers, for the benefit of avoidance of repeated medication. The implementation of zero mark-up policy cancelled the differential between purchase and sale price of EMs. And a fiscal management approach called separation of revenue and expenditure budgets (SREB) was recommended to implement. It was public PHIs that had to turn in their all revenue, and government financial sectors would make an overall plan of appropriation according to PHIs' actual and reasonable needs. These measures were expected to eliminate perverse economic incentives to avert excessive use of medicines. However, the mechanism of financial compensation for public health institutions was defective, resulting in reduction of health workers' enthusiasm and PHIs' performance, unmet demand for medicines use in PHCs, poor delivery efficiency etc. They could also generate negative impact to RUM. (Yu et al., 2011)

In addition to the NEMS, there are also a wide range of regulations and policies to guide RUM, such as Drug Administration Law, Prescription Regulation,

---

① Source: WHO database on medicines use 2009.

Pharmaceutical Administration for Health Institutions etc., which generally or specifically stipulate clinical medicine use, and Chinese Pharmacopeia, Chinese National Formulary, Clinical Medication Guidelines of National Essential Medicines, Clinical Medication Guidelines for Physicians and Pharmacists etc. which provide health workers and patients with professional knowledge and instructive information of health and medicine based on pharmacoeconomics, evidence-based medicines (EBM), pharmacoepidemiology and so on. (Guan & Shi, 2009b)

Across the nation, various regions have their own strategies to promote RUM. Local health workers take part in formulating and improving the standard of clinical treatment, and the standard is distributed to the mass with introduction and training and will be amended according to prescription review and feedback. The NEMS handbook is formulated by local institutions, distributed to the mass with training, and revised according to investigation on medicine use. Hospital pharmaceutical administration unit is established to enact interior formulary and STGs, assess medicine use and control nosocomial infection, educate and train physicians and pharmacists, manage the effect caused by medicine sales promotion, monitor and prevent ADR and misuse of medicines, and provide the management of medicine quality and the counsel of cost control. Local institutions develop training of diagnosis and treatment for common frequently-encountered diseases as well as medicine use, and diffuse RUM concept. Medicine experts review and supervise medicine use, and hospitals investigate prescriptions and provide feedback. Independent information system is established to dispatch medicine information provided by CFDA, MoH etc. in hospitals. Public education of medication is launched to disseminate knowledge of RUM, e.g. benefit of the NEMS, and treatment for common diseases to drug retailers, patients and the public by printed materials and electronic media. Economic measures include disconnecting physicians' income with the quantity of prescribed medicines, and reimbursing the expense only if the case passes the medical record censor and the medicine use is not beyond a restrict list. Institutional construction is also pushed forward by medicine regulators, including medicine supply regulation, such as centralized public bidding in medicine purchasing and supply assurance, stringent supervision for prescription medicines, strict admittance management for medicine distributors, contract administration on normal medicine use, institutionalized and standardized management of RUM, change in payment to control the medicine expense, and SREB in primary health institutions. Government investment is ensured to raise the efficiency of medication and treatment, in terms of increasing hospital financial investment and health workers' revenue, putting medical security funding in place, and reimbursing expenses of medicines in the EML or the insured medicine directory. (Yang, 2006)

2.5 NEMS and RUM

2.5.1 Concept of NEMS and the related

According to WHO, EMs are those that satisfy the priority health care needs of the population. They are selected with due regard to public health relevance, evidence on efficacy and safety, and comparative cost-effectiveness. EMs are intended to be available within the context of functioning health systems at all times in adequate amounts, in the appropriate dosage forms, with assured quality and adequate information, and at a price the individual and the community can afford. (WHO/DAP, 1998)

NEMS is a systematic national medicine policy on many aspects, such as development, manufacture, distribution, prescribing, and use of EMs with code of guidance, implementation measures as well as supervision and regulation, in order to ensure the satisfaction of public, improve availability, accessibility, affordability and rational use of EMs, allocate the health resources rationally, harmonize the relationship among medical service, medication and fundamental health security system effectively. (Meng, 2009)

EML is a global health strategy promoted by WHO and the core component of NEMS. The medicines in the list have been evaluated scientifically and selected in accordance with the spectrum of disease and the socio-economic development with evidence-based method. EML aims to select medicines with credible safety, reliable efficacy, faithful quality and fair price, and meet the basic health needs. EML could also serve as a reference for medicine purchasing, supply and donation, medicine expenditure reimbursement, and pharmaceutical manufacture. (Laing et al., 2003).

STGs, also called treatment protocols or clinical guidelines, are systematically developed statements that assist prescribers in deciding on appropriate treatment for specific conditions. (Tett, 2004) By using STGs, prescribing practices can be rationalized and patient outcomes can be improved, along with the optimum use of the limited resources for medicines. Together with an EML, STGs are powerful tools in promoting RUM, and they are integral in strategies to reduce antimicrobial resistance. (Grimshaw et al., 2004) Now there are more than 120 STGs formulated by WHO, covering the treatment for malaria, HIV/AIDS, tuberculosis, cancer, diabetes, and so on.

NF specifies particular medications that are approved for prescription throughout the country, indicating which products are interchangeable. It includes key information on the composition, description, selection, prescribing, dispensing and administration of medicines. In most developing countries, the NF is limited to medicines on the national EML. WHO enacted its model formulary in 2002.

2.5.2 History of NEMS

2.5.2.1 Budding stage (1959-1974)

In the 1960s and 1970s, most diseases could have an effective treatment, though the efficacy was less than desirable. However, due to low health investment, lack of health facilities and staff, backward drug supply system and high drug cost, people in poverty were unable to access or afford the medicines they need. Meanwhile, irrational use of medicines made medications low effective or void. At that time, there was very little objective information regarding RUM and no public information about drug price. Only a very few countries advocated generic drugs as alternatives. (WHO, 2010a) Since 1959, Ceylon (now known as Sri Lanka), Peru, Tanzania etc. had attempted to draft an EML in order to address the most urgent demand for medicines. (Mamdani, 1992)

2.5.2.2 Initial stage (1975-1984)

In 1975, the 28th World Health Assembly (WHA), held in Geneva, requested WHO to assist developing countries selecting and purchasing medicines with super quality and competitive price, and the concept of EMs and national medicines policy were first proposed and soon afterwards accepted by global public health circle. In the October of 1977, WHO Technical Report Series No. 615 formally formulated the concept of EMs as medicines that satisfied the priority health care needs for most of the population. Meanwhile, WHO took action plan for the selection of EMs as its strategic mission, and put out the first model EML. (WHO, 2002a) In 1978, The Declaration of Almaty identified "provision of EMs" as one of the eight elements of PHC, which was a crucial milestone of global public health. (WHO/UNICEF, 1978) WHO/DAP was founded in 1981, and the concept of EMs was developed.

2.5.2.3 Developmental stage (1985-1998)

WHO developed EMs strategy in the 1985 Nairobi conference, stressing EMs procurement, distribution, quality assurance and especially rational use beyond selection into the list, and pointed out their validity for developed countries. (WHO, 1987) In 1991, a review on WHO's essential medicines policy spoke highly of the increment of generic medicines out of essential medicines, and proposed that information of comparative cost of those in EML should be provided. (Howard & Laing, 1991) WHO and MSH jointly introduced how to select essential medicines according to the prevalence of diseases and existing STGs in 1997, in order to promote the standardization and normalization of diagnosis and medication. (Quick et al., 1997) More and more countries and international organizations adopted the concept of EMs, WHO model list and national medicines policy in this period.

2.5.2.4 Mature stage (from 1999 to today)

In 1999, WHO published a manual to guide and demonstrate how to monitor national medicines policy. In the same year, when WHO expert committee amended the EML, they believed that evidence supporting was needed and there needed a synopsis of evidence for review. (WHO, 2000b) Between 2000 and 2001, the criterions of selection for EML changed a lot, of which the most significant one was that evidence-based selection was adopted instead of experience-based selection. (WHO/EDM, 2001) Doha Declaration on TRIPS (Agreement on Trade-Related Aspects of Intellectual Property Rights) and Public Health 2001 made it clear that public health was prior to patent rights when it came to medicine, in order to protect the countries who were incapable to produce the medicines they need, mitigate the procedural barriers to international distribution of medicines, and promote EMs availability for various countries. (Hoen, 2002) In 2002, WHO made an accurate statement to essential medicines from essential drugs, and finalized the concept of EMs as today, including efficacy, safety, adaptability to PHC needs and cost-effectiveness. (WHO, 2002c)

Nowadays, NEMS has driven to maturity by focusing on the following three issues : (1) availability and affordability, to improve the supply chain, to eliminate knowledge, economy and institution barriers, and to make people capable to pay for the EMs; (2) RUM, to monitor the use of EMs and to intervene the behaviors of health workers; (3) quality, to ensure safety, efficacy and stability of EMs, and to enforce pharmacovigilance. (WHO, 2010b)

2.5.3 Country experiences

2.5.3.1 Delhi Paradigm in India

Delhi State, the capital of India, first introduced EMs programme in 1994, which was a set of measures for the implementation of the NEMS and RUM policy. The objectives of the programme are to improve the availability, accessibility and affordability of EMs, including 10 contents: (1) Selection of an EML; (2) Establishment of a pooled procurement system; (3) Preparation of formulary; (4) Introduction of a quality assurance system; (5) Training in rational prescribing; (6) Provision of drug information (to doctors and for patient guidance); (7) Development of standard treatment guidelines; (8) Contents of drug advertising and promotion; (9) Research on implementation of drug policy; (10) Monitoring and evaluation on EMs and RUM. (*Drug Policy of the National Capital Territory of Delhi*, 1994) The government works in close collaboration with the Delhi Society for the Promotion of Rational Use of Drugs (DSPRUD) and university experts to implement the policy effectively. With those measures, medicines price in Delhi has dropped by 30%, and RUM has been substantially improved. Delhi paradigm was promoted by WHO as a successful story of PHC program. (Chaudhury et al., 2005)

The EML was developed by a committee consisting of a cross-disciplinary group of physicians, pharmacists, microbiologists, production technicians and other experts. The EML comprises two parts, for outpatient use and inpatient use, and is amended annually. As for the regulation, to ensure efficacy of the EML and use of the EMs, the off-list medicine cost must account for no more than 10% of the total medicine cost in general hospitals and 20% in special hospitals. (Guan & Shi, 2009a)

The procurement, storage and distribution of EMs are in centralized supervision by state Centralized Procurement Agency. Only those in the list could be procured based on competitive bidding through tenders. Two Envelop Selective Tender System (TESTS) is implemented in the course of procurement. Technical parameters and price quote are enclosed in two separate envelops, and only if the technical standard is met, the quote will be considered. In order to ensure the safety and efficacy of the medicines coming to users, measures for quality control and quality assurance are implemented, including GMP compliance as well as laboratory inspection and control in production, and recall of non-compliant medicines timely in distribution.

With the purpose of promotion of RUM, STGs and model formulary are also enacted, advantaging control on medicine cost, delivery of norm of treatment, as well as specification of health workers' behavior for diagnosis and treatment. The RUM training is open for physicians, pharmacists and medicine storage keepers regularly, and the latest medicine information is periodically released to the public. To ensure that the proper information is delivered, medicine advertisement and promotion are stringently regulated. In addition, monitoring, assessment and research on EMs and RUM are carried out in case of any needs for intervention. (Liu, Qian & Zhang, 2003)

2.5.3.2　Kenya

Kenya has always been the foregoer of essential medicines policy since the 1980s. Kenya has modified its medicine supply system roundly with the measures as below: (1) establishing a medicine registration system; (2) procuring medicines by generic names; (3) procuring and using those in the EML; (4) budgeting a reasonable medicine requirement; (5) validating the qualification of medicine suppliers; (6) monitoring medicine suppliers' behavior; (7) ensuring and optimizing the medicine distribution. (Kenya MMS & Kenya MPHS, 2009)

In the aspect of improving affordability, canonical prescriptions and alternative medicines stressed. Dissemination of generic medicines to physicians, pharmacists, other health workers and the public is enhanced to acquire recognition of economy and efficacy of generic medicines. Medicine price information is released periodically and exchanged with other nations. The coverage of National Hospital Insurance Fund (NHIF) and other medical insurance are expanded to mitigate economic burden of medication in order to contain as many medicines as possible in the list.

In the respect of RUM, Kenya promotes up-to-date STGs to hospitals and clinics in countryside, involve the concept of EMs and RUM in medical training courses, establish a committee of pharmaceuticals and therapeutics and a national medicine information system, and encourage use of EMs prescribed in generic names. (Ogendi, 2011)

2.5.3.3 Australia

Australia has emerged over the past two decades as a world leader in medicine policy. Its national drug strategy has been characterized by a unique combination of features which have brought it international attention and acclaim. (Norman, 2001) National Medicines Policy (NMP), introduced in 2000, is to overcome adversarial relations between key stakeholders and to ensure equitable access to safe and efficacious medicines of good quality. It has contributed to a variety of groups including state agencies, the pharmaceutical industry, health practitioners, consumers and other interests. Four pivotal objectives are identified: (1) timely access to the medicines that Australians need, at a cost individuals and the community can afford; (2) medicines meeting adequate criterion of safety, efficacy and quality; (3) quality use of medicines; and (4) maintaining a liable and viable medicine industry. (Lofgren & Boer, 2004)

Australia has a well-developed process for the appraisal and listing of medicines. During the 1980s, Australia embraced the use of EBM, and in 1992 Australia became the first country in the world to bring in CEA and CBA of medicines as a mandatory requirement before listing on the Pharmaceutical Benefits Schedule (PBS). Medicines on the PBS are subsidized by the Australian government for all Australians, while those that are not listed on the PBS may be publicly funded through statewide formularies or hospitals. By the means of limitation of reimbursement from the universal health insurance and control of EMs cost, the medicine price in Australia is much lower than that in Europe.

Australia formulates a proper, safe and rational medication strategy and constitutes a national formulary office, whose responsibility is publishing STG and medicines handbook to standardize physicians' behavior, engaging on academic promotion to provide prescription information for physicians, offering training program to medics, junior physicians and nurses. With the measures rich in contents and with multitudinousness, RUM has been promoted in the round. (Shen, 2003)

2.5.3.4　Summary of implications

According to these three countries' experiences, promoting RUM is embodied in the concept of EMs, and the measures are stressed as one of the pivotal. Health workers' awareness and understanding of RUM and EMs are essential to their behaviors, which also need to be standardized and normalized by STGs or other policies. Centralized procurement and distribution are attested effective to ensure medicines supply. Also, Australia's experience on selection of medicines into the list based on evidence and cost-effectiveness analysis is a very precious direction for any countries with sufficient information to conduct related studies to improve economical efficiency of medication.

2.5.4　The NEMS of China

2.5.4.1　Evolution of NEMS

China involved actively in the Action Programme on Essential Drugs when NEMS was initially proposed and when it was being promoted to developing countries by WHO. In April 1979, National Essential Medicines Selection Group was founded and engaged in formulating China's first EML, which was accomplished in August 1981 and launched in January of the following year. The concept of EMs was first introduced to China then, but there was not any supporting institutional measures.

During the two decades between the 1980s and the early 2000s, EML evolved along with the reform of the medical insurance system. (Huang, 2007) With the development of economy under the context of reform and opening-up policy, the old health care system was unable to afford the health needs. Labor medical care system had been gradually eliminated since the 1990s and medical insurance for urban workers was established in 1998. Meanwhile, massive medicines were traded in the market without adequate administration of manufacturing, distribution and clinical use, resulting in the shortage of medicines and bogus or substandard medicines influx in hospitals. EMs related policies and basic medical insurance system can assort with each other, covering more people, curbing the pace of rise in health expenditures, and improving medicine distribution. (Han, Gao & Shen, 2008). Between January 1992 and December 1994, China was designated as the delegate of the WHO/DAP Regional Office for the Western Pacific (WPRO). National Essential Medicines Leading Group was established in 1992 to formulate policies and guidelines as well as the list of essential medicines, and coordinate the planning and implementation of NEMS. EMs were selected based on "clinical requirement, safety and efficacy, reasonable price and convenience", as a reference of reimbursement for socialized medical services. At the same time, the government busted a gut to ensure manufacturing and supply of EMs on demand. (China MoH, 1992) Between 1996 and 2004, there were 5 versions of EML published (see Table 2-2). (Yu, 2007)

Table 2-2　　Number of varieties of medicines in successive EMLs of China

Years of Version	1982	1996	1998	2000	2002	2004	2009	2012
Chemical or Biological Medicines	278	699	740	770	759	773	205	317
TCMs	N/A	1,812	1,570	1,249	1,242	1,260	102	203

During this period, national essential medicines policy of China was coordinated with the medical security system reform as a supplement. Thus, a systematic NEMS was not established, resulting in poor practicality of EMs and EML. As the medical insurance system for urban workers was completely constituted and the medicine list for national basic medical insurance and employment injury insurance was widely adopted, so that EML gradually faded.

2.5.4.2　The NEMS under the context of the NHCR

From 2006 to 2007, China went through a new round health care reform, "establishing the NEMS, to rectify the order in the field of medicine manufacturing and distribution, and to ensure medicine supply to meet people's basic needs" (Chen, Ye, Ying & Jiang, 2007). The NHCR was formally launched on April 6, 2009. Five key reform projects were: (1) accelerating the construction of the basic medical security system, which shall completely cover urban and rural residents; (2) preliminarily establishing a national essential medicines system for the selection, production and supply, use and reimbursement of essential medicines through medical insurance; (3) improving the grassroots health care services system; (4) promoting the progressive equalization of the basic public health services; and (5) promoting the pilot reform on public hospitals. (CPC Central Comittee & State Council, 2009)

The NEMS aims to improve medicine availability and affordability, thus to achieve the goal of everybody enjoying the primary health care with limited funds and resources. On August 18 of the same year, three documents: Opinions on Establishing National Essential Medicine System, Measures for the Administration of National Essential Medicines List (Tentative) and National Essential Medicines List (for Grassroots Health Institutions Use) were released, which marked the official initiation of the NEMS of China. The EML 2009 consisted of 307 medicines, of which 205 were chemical or biological medicines and 102 were traditional Chinese medicines (TCMs) (see Table 2-2), and they were divided into over 20 common therapeutic categories. With the implementation of the NHCR and supporting policies, this EML got legal force somewhat, conducive to the effective regulation and steering on EMs manufacturing, distribution and use, and as the basis of outfit and use of medicines in health institutions. Since then, EMs in China has been not only a concept, but also an effective public policy.

The major measures of the NEMS are highlighted as the following:

(1) Selection. Scope and principle for selection of EMs are stipulated by the selection protocol, and EML is subject to modify every three years. In addition, provincial governments are authorized to formulate their own provincial supplementary essential medicines lists (PEMLs) so as to address

local medical needs. Those listed in PEML are regulated as EMs in the specific province.

(2)Production. EMs must be manufactured under the guideline of GMP. CFDA monitors EMs by a standard barcode attached to the package of EMs electronically.

(3)Procurement and distribution. Public health institutions purchase EMs through provincial centralized procurement systems under the rule of online public bidding. EMs should be delivered integratedly by qualified enterprises with modern logistic capability.

(4)Utilization. PHIs should outfit EMs and those listed in PEML, and use them following STGs and NF. Secondary and tertiary hospitals are encouraged to use EMs as priority.

(5)Pricing. Zero mark-up policy is implemented within PHIs, with no profit for the sale of EMs. Maximum retail prices of EMs were set by National Development and Reform Commission (NDRC), but this policy has not been applicable to most medicines since June, 2015.

(6)Reimbursement. All EMs are covered by social medical insurance, and reimbursed at a higher rate than non-list medicines.

The EML 2009 along with the supporting policies played a vital role in promoting RUM, mitigating the economic burden on patients and building a new operation mechanism of PHIs. However, there were some limitations during the implementation: narrow variety of medicines resulting in dissatisfaction of EMs in PHIs and underuse of EMs in secondary and tertiary hospitals; insufficient medicines specialized in maternity, pediatrics, oncology and so on; unstandardized supplementary medicines list; broad dosage form and administration dose going against procurement with quantity. Based on the EML 2009, the latest version of EML was released in 2012, a total of 520 medicines with 317 chemical or biological medicines and 203 TCMs (see Table 2-2). The variety of medicines was added to fulfill the PHC needs and to make EMs applicable to the patients in advanced health institutions for priority of use. The therapeutic categories were optimized, as for the prevalence of the common diseases, especially the serious medical conditions, and the demographics. The EML 2012 was put into a standard model for easy monitoring and regulation of medicines use, and corresponded to the basic health insurance programs for convenient and high-proportion reimbursement. (China NHFPC，2012)

A large number of literatures have assessed and reviewed the effectiveness and problems of the NEMS. Song's (2013) study conducted in four provinces discovers that median price of medicines decreased by more or less 1/3 within one or two years after the NEMS was launched，but was still higher than international reference price (IRP). Decrease of price also led to the new shortage of some medicines and substantial financial losses faced with by most PHIs while compensation for this reduction was largely ineffective. Availability of EMs reached 2/3 in PHIs by 2011. Use of EMs was improved，and over-prescription of antibiotics and injections as well as poly-pharmacy remained common. In addition，93. 31% of patients and 92. 54% of PHI staff were satisfied with the NEMS. Song believes that the NEMS has achieved positive effect on RUM，but there remain negative outcomes that requires further policy design and implementation. A research on 522 PHIs of 26 provinces also finds evident decrease of medicine price and average prescription fee，continuous improvement of RUM，shortage and quality issues of some EMs，and financial deficit of some PHIs. The study also indicates the regional discrepancy of status and effect of the NEMS implementation：the overall achievement in eastern region was obviously better than that in the central region and western region. Socio-economic status can significantly affect the availability and affordability of EMs as well as the institutional development of PHIs. (Cao，2014) Another study involving 40% of CHCs nationwide reports the similar results. (Li，2011)

Tang (1998) believes that promoting RUM is imperative and essential for the NEMS under the NHCR, and the effort to bridge the gap of the NEMS，PHC and RUM should be made to strongly support the policy implementation and achieve intended impact.

2. 6　The SDUIs

2. 6. 1　WHO/INRUD manual for medicine use

A medicine use study usually has one or more of these goals：describing existing medication practices, comparing the performance of individual institutions and/or prescribers, monitoring and supervising specific medicine use behaviors periodically, and/or evaluating the impact of an intervention by using indicators.

WHO/INRUD released How to Investigate Drug Use in Medical Facilities: Selected Drug Use Indicators in 1993, setting forth a set of indicators for health facilities to assess RUM. 3 groups of 12 core indicators and another 7 complementary indicators were proposed for both outpatients and inpatients, including prescribing indicators, patient care indicators, health facility indicators, etc. (see Table 2-3) (WHO, 1993) Not only does the SDUIs contain medicine utilization information, but also it involves humanity concern over physicians' and pharmacists' service, so as to evaluate the medicine therapy status scientifically and impartially in a health institution. (Chen, 2011)

Table 2-3　　　　　　　　**Selected drug use indicators**

Core Indicators	
Prescribing indicators	
1	Average number of drugs per encounter
2	Percentage of drugs prescribed by generic name
3	Percentage of encounters with an antibiotic prescribed
4	Percentage of encounters with an injection prescribed
5	Percentage of drugs prescribed from essential drug list or formulary
Patient care indicators	
6	Average consultation time
7	Average dispensing time
8	Percentage of drugs actually dispensed
9	Percentage of drugs adequately labelled
10	Patients' knowledge of correct usage
Health facility indicators	
11	Availability of copy of essential drugs list or formulary
12	Availability of key drugs
Complementary Indicators	

Continued

13	Percentage of patients treated without drugs
14	Average drug cost per encounter
15	Percentage of drug costs spent on antibiotics
16	Percentage of drug costs spent on injections
17	Prescription in accordance with treatment guidelines
18	Percentage of patients satisfied with the care they received
19	Percentage of health facilities with access to impartial drug information

Core indicators are highly standardized with no need for national or regional adaption, and are highly recommended in any medicine use studies. These provide a simple, quick and reliable tool to evaluate some pivotal issues of medicine use in health institutions. The prescription indicators are the kernel of the core indicators, which scale the performance of prescribers regarding appropriate use of medicines, based on the observation of clinical practices by collecting encounter records (see Table 2-4). Patient care indicators evaluate the medicine use in health facilities from patient's perspectives, managing patients experience in health institutions and interaction between health workers and patients to observe potential quality limits on diagnosis and treatment. Facility indicators are able to reflect the characteristics of the environment in health institutions that can influence rational prescribing behaviors. Complementary indicators are as important as core indicators, but are more difficult to obtain or highly sensitive to local settings with restrained reliability. (WHO, 1993)

Table 2-4　　　　　**Meanings of SDUIs prescribing indicators**

Indicators	Meanings
Average number of drugs per encounter	Reflect the basic situation of medicine use and polypharmacy, so as to evaluate the degree of overuse of medicines
Percentage of drugs prescribed by generic name	Operating standardization indicators, prescribing with generic name are beneficial to avoidance the of errors, reflecting health workers' skills and ability

Continued

Indicators	Meanings
Percentage of encounters with an antibiotic prescribed	Illustrate the extent of antibiotics use, providing preliminary data of polypharmacy and RUM
Percentage of encounters with an injection prescribed	Reflect overuse of injections, evaluating improper application of dosage form
Percentage of drugs prescribed from essential drug list of formulary	Preliminarily evaluate the degree of outfit and promotion of EMs

The SDUIs, which is an objective and scientific analytic technique and research model, was built on the early systematic studies on evaluating the effect of NEMS conducted in Yemen and Uganda. (Christensen, 1990; Hogerzeil et al., 1989) Hereafter, the researchers who are engaged in investigating medicine use in developing countries have adopted this method. The indicators are not always entirely used in the studies, of which many apply part of SDUIs and/or modified some indicators based on their study design and data collection. (Bashrahil, 2010; Odusanya, 2004)

In 2007, WHO released an operational package that described a systematic method for assessing the medicine situation, including access to and rational use of quality medicines. It builds a 3-level-core-indicator hierarchical approach to systematically measure the most essential details to draw a comprehensive landscape of medicine situation in a country. Among the core indicators, the Level II indicators provide systematic data on access and rational use of quality medicines, which correspond to the SDUIs (see Table 2-5). By providing specific data about important medicine outcomes to support the Level I indicators that provide rapid means of retrieving information on the current infrastructure and key processes of each component of the pharmaceutical sector, and along with Level III indicators that list more details of the components, these indicators can assess the capacity of a country, such as available infrastructure, logistics and human resources to support the pharmaceutical sector and implement national medicines policies; monitor the implementation of medicines policies; measure the impact of implementation strategies; and evaluate progress towards identified objectives. (WHO, 2007b)

Table 2-5   Level II facility core outcome indicators in WHO hierarchical approach—rational use of medicines

1	Percentage of medicines adequately labelled at public health facility dispensaries and private drug outlets
2	Percentage of patients knowing how to take medicines at public health facility dispensaries and private drug outlets
3	Average number of medicines per prescription at public health facility dispensaries and private drug outlets
4	Percentage of patients prescribed antibiotics in public health facilities
5	Percentage of patients prescribed injections in public health facilities
6	Percentage of prescribed medicines on the essential medicine list at public health facilities
7	Percentage of medicines prescribed by generic name at public health facilities
8	Availability of essential medicine list at public health facilities
9	Availability of standard treatment guidelines at public health facilities
10	Percentage of tracer cases treated according to recommended treatment protocol/guide at public health facilities
11	Percentage of prescription medicines bought with no prescription

2. 6. 2   WHO reference values for SDUIs

For years, WHO has been devoted to the advocacy and promotion of RUM research and practice, especially in the third world countries.

How to Investigate Drug Use in Medical Facilities: Selected Drug Use Indicators sets forth that on average 2-3 medicines per encounter was appropriate for grassroots health institutions in rural areas, and provides the survey indicators from 11 Asian and African countries (see Table 2-6). (WHO, 1993) Moreover, in 1997, WHO derived standard values of the indicators for outpatient medicine use in health institutions of developing countries (see Table 2-7). (Tang et al., 1998)

Table 2-6　　　Survey indicators from 11 Asian and African countries

Indicators	Range
Average number of drugs per encounter	1. 3-3. 8
Percentage of drugs prescribed by generic name	37-94
Percentage of encounters with an antibiotic prescribed	27-63
Percentage of encounters with an injection prescribed	0. 2-48
Percentage of drugs prescribed from essential drug list or formulary	86-88
Average consultation time (minute)	2. 3-6. 3
Average dispensing time (second)	12. 5-86. 1
Percentage of drugs actually dispensed	70-83
Patients' knowledge of correct usage	27-82
Availability of key drugs	38-90

Table 2-7　　　　　WHO reference values for SDUIs

Indicators	WHO Standard Value	Ideal Value
Average number of medicines per encounter	1. 6-2. 8	<2
Percentage of medicines prescribed by generic name	100	100. 0
Percentage of medicines prescribed from essential medicine list of formulary	100	100. 0
Percentage of encounters with an antibiotic prescribed	20. 0-26. 7	$<30. 0$
Percentage of encounters with an injection prescribed	13. 4-24. 1	$<20. 0$

In March, 2004, WHO held the Second International Conference on Improving Use of Medicines, and the conventioneers agreed that there was much research gap of the criterion of the indicators. (Wang, Wang & Ma, 2004) The observed values in 35 countries in this year were shown in Table 2-8.

Table 2-8   Observed values of the indicators in 35 Countries (2004)

Indicators	Observed Value
Average number of medicines per encounter	2.39
Percentage of encounters with antibiotics prescribed	44.8
Percentage of encounters with injections prescribed	22.8

In 2006, WHO monitored the indicators from 57 low-income countries and 65 middle-income countries, with values shown in Table 2-2-9.

Table 2-9   Observed values in WHO monitoring (2006)

Indicators	Observed Values in WHO Monitoring	
	Median(Q1, Q3) of 57 low-income countries	Median (Q1, Q3) of 65 middle-income countries
Average number of medicines per encounter	2.7(2.2-2.9)	2.5(2.4-3.0)
Percentage of encounters with antibiotics prescribed	51.7(45.0-60.0)	43.3(36.7-50.0)
Percentage of encounters with injections prescribed	23.1(11.3-28.8)	6.7(0-10.5)

2.6.3   The SDUIs application in China

The SDUIs was introduced into China in 1995. (Tang et al., 1995) Between February and October in 2001, CFDA carried out a series of multi-center investigations on RUM by using SDUIs under the guidance of WHO officials and experts. Wang et al.(2002) evaluates and compares the status of medicine use across hospitals by SDUIs, and results show the effectiveness, feasibility and adequacy of the indicators for investigation on RUM in China. After that, more and more studies involved SDUIs to investigate medicine use. Numerous researches were conducted in an attempt to evaluate the effect of the NEMS on RUM under the context of the NHCR in recent years. The prescription indicators were most frequently applied in these studies, most of which were of special concern on antibiotics use and some of which involved the patient care indicators as well as the facility indicators. (Li, Li & Yang, 2011)

Zhang & Zheng(2005) studies the reference range for the value of the RUM indicators in the rural areas of China by literature review. Not only do they point out that the prescription indicators was placed extra emphasis on and the patient care indicators as well as the facility indicators were usually omitted, but also they find that the prescription indicators was relatively high and the facility indicators was relatively low compared to the WHO results.

Yan et al. (2005) conducts a sampling survey on outpatient prescriptions to investigate the RUM by the SDUIs in six secondary public hospitals in Shanghai suburb in 2004, which shows that the average number of medicines per encounter was 2.7, the percentage of encounters with an antibiotic prescribed was 43%, the percentage of encounters with an injection prescribed was 25.4%, the percentage of medicines prescribed from the EML was 66.6%, the average consultation time was 8.67 minutes, the average dispensing time was 24.9 seconds, the percentage of medicines adequately labelled was 89.2%, the patients' knowledge of correct usage was 88.3%, and the percentage of patients satisfied with the care they received was 79.2%. (Yan et al., 2005)

Guan et al. (2007) used SDUIs to investigate outpatient medicine use with the prescriptions within six months in a tertiary hospital in Shanghai in 2006, indicating that the average number of medicines per outpatient prescription was 2.15, the percentage of encounters with an antibiotic prescribed was 24.68%, the percentage of encounters with an injection prescribed was 10.25%, the percentage of the EMs prescribed was 97.4%; the average consultation time was 3.8 minutes, the average dispensing time was 25 seconds, the percentage of medicines actually dispensed reached 100%, the percentage of medicines adequately labelled was 95%, and the patients' knowledge of correct usage was 85%.

Dong et al. (2011) developed an index for rational drug prescribing (IRDP) based on some of the indicators by applying a mathematical model for comprehensive appraisal and used it to measure medicine prescribing in 680 VHCs from 40 counties in 10 provinces of western China. The average number of medicines per prescription was 2.36, while the percentage of medicines prescribed by generic name was 64.12% and the percentage of medicines prescribed from the EML was 67.70%. 48.43% and 22.93% of the total prescriptions contained antibiotics and injections respectively. The IRDP was 3.32 out of the optimal level 5. Overuse of antibiotics and injections were the most remarkable characteristics of the irrational medicine prescribing.

Kuang et al. (2014) investigates medicine use with the prescription indicators and the patient care indicators in a secondary hospital in 2012. The average number of medicines prescribed per encounter was 3.26, the percentage of prescriptions including antibiotics and injections were 23.73% and 16.38% respectively, the percentage of prescriptions using the EMs was 27.78%, the percentage of medicines prescribed by generic name was 100%, and the average medicine cost per capita was 167.81 *yuan* The average consultation time was 8.45 minutes, the average dispensing time was 28.50 seconds, the percentage of medicines actually dispensed and medicines adequately labelled achieved 100%, and the patients' knowledge of correct usage was 87%. The results shows that most indicators in this study was rational, but polypharmacy, high medicine cost, low utilization rate of EMs, as well as lack of patient cares were the problems.

Zhang et al. (2014) studies the impact of NEMS on RUM. They investigates prescriptions spanning 3 years over the time point of NEMS launch from THCs in Ningxia, indicating that the effect on use of antibiotics and injections were limited. They also tries to add the percentage of prescriptions with hormone use as RUM indicators.

Wei and Zeng (2016) carries out a study on outpatient RUM and related factors in a tertiary hospital in Shenzhen in 2015. They discover that the proportion of EMs use was low, while use of antibiotics and injections were effectively controlled. Prescribers' technical title and working experience were the two positive factors affecting the RUM.

The SDUIs were widely used in the researches on medicine use in China.

Chapter 3　Methodology

3. 1　Research objectives

RUM in the vast rural areas concerns the health of three quarters of the Chinese population, and is an essential public issue of rural PHC which the NHCR pledges an endeavor to improve. Researches on medicine utilization there are helpful for approaching medicines safely, effectively and economically for rural residents. The general objective is to investigate the outpatient medicine use under the context of the NHCR in rural areas of China, monitoring the status of RUM, and to identify the organizational barriers of health institutions on the achievement of RUM by establishing a comprehensive evaluation method for RUM outcomes. It also attempts to provide some policy recommendations and suggestive strategies based on the results.

The specific objectives are:

(1) To evaluate the effect of the NEMS on RUM;

(2) To appraise the status of RUM when the NEMS becomes mature and the NHCR is at the in-depth stage;

(3) To attempt to establish a comprehensive evaluation method for RUM outcomes;

(4) To identify the obstructive factors regarding health organizations that influence the achievement of RUM.

3.2 Research design

For Objective (1), a pre and post comparative analysis is designed during two time periods before and after the implementation of the NEMS. This longitudinal study can obtain more concentrated data and is applied to causality analysis that is adequate for evaluating the effect of the NEMS on RUM. Cross-sectional study is not suitable for this for the following two reasons. Firstly, The NEMS rolled out rapidly throughout the whole country within one year. Each province declared to enforce the NEMS, and the NEMS was implemented in the PHIs in one geographic unit at almost the same time. Thus, it is impossible to divide the sample sites into interventional group and control group for parallel design. Secondly, socio-economic development, as well as local regulation and policy details, varies greatly across the regions, resulting in exceeding difficulty in controlling the confounding factors. The projected analysis with trend line is not applicable as well, because the medicine policy in China changed a lot in the previous years and the policy details adjusted frequently in the later period, so the periods of both pre and post implementation of the NEMS are not long enough for the analysis. In addition, PHIs are the selected sites for this analysis, because the NEMS focuses on basic medication needs and was initiated in the PHIs at the early stage.

For Objective (2), a cross-sectional study involving much more sites is employed. The NEMS becomes mature and the policies gets stable after 2012, so it is better to involve more health facilities as the observed subjects across various regions to fully reflect the existing status of RUM under the context of NHCR.

For Objective (3), by using the raw data and the results for the Objective (2), principal component analysis (PCA) is used to establish a comprehensive evaluation index of RUM based on the SDUIs. Multiple variables make study complicated, and to obtain more information with fewer variables brings about simple and convenient analysis. PCA is a simple, well-developed and frequently used approach of multivariate analysis for dimensionality reduction to provide an explicit scene of the data that tell the story of targeted project by extracting fewer new variables from the original variables that may be correlated and repeated. (Shaw, 2003)

For Objective (4), a multivariate regression analysis is applied. The comprehensive evaluation index of RUM derived from the previous stage of this research is used as an outcome indicator, and organizational barriers associated with the achievement of RUM of a health institution are identified as influential factors. The organizational factors include institution setting, manpower support, as well as funding structure and fiscal incentives. (Yang et al., 2015) A health institution is the physical site and the basic element to implement the medicine policies, so to explore the impediments to smooth effectuation, discovering the concrete issues, by a single organization is a faithful way to understand the feasibility and the sustainability of the policies that promote RUM, hence to propose some viable and reliable measures to improve the enforcement of RUM related policies and regulations.

3.3 Data source

Data were collected by undertaking several field surveys by our project team as well as some partnership organizations.

3.3.1 First hand data from field study

Four provinces (Zhejiang, Anhui, Shandong and Ningxia) with different socio-economic status were selected as study regions to carry out field study on the effect of the NEMS on RUM. Zhejiang and Shandong are representatives of the richest inshore provinces located in eastern China, Anhui is in the central China with moderate development, and Ningxia is a less developed in northwestern area of China. Calculated by dividing the regional gross domestic product (GDP) by the local population, GDP per capita of Zhejiang, Anhui, Shandong and Ningxia in 2009 were RMB 43575.34, 16413.02, 35793.72 and 21652.96 *yuan* respectively, and the rank of GDP per capita for these four areas remained unchanged from 2009 to 2011.

The data from Zhejiang and Anhui were collected through the program "Mid-term Evaluation on Implementation Effect of Essential Medicines Policy" organized by NDRC in the end of 2010. The program was conducted in 12 counties of 4 prefecture cities, Hangzhou and Shaoxing in Zhejiang and Hefei and Bengbu in Anhui, 3 counties for each prefecture city respectively, which were selected with stratified sampling, and involved 139 PHIs in total.

The data from Shandong and Ningxia were collected by our project team through cooperative efforts with local academic institutions and government agencies in 2011. The on-site survey in Shandong was conducted in Ju County involving all 21 PHIs, and in Ningxia the investigation was carried out in 16 PHIs, of which 8 was in Xiji county, 4 was in Tongxin county and the other 4 was in Qingtongxia county (see Table 3-1).

Table 3-1   Quantity and distribution of PHIs in the field study
on the effect of the NEMS on RUM

	No. of PHIs	Time span of the data
Zhejiang	99	2009-2010
Anhui	40	
Shandong	21	2010-2011
Ningxia	16	
Total	176	

3.3.2 Secondary data from CMB project

China Medical Board (CMB) launched a large project named "Situational Analysis and Policy Evaluation of Deployment and Retention of Human Resources for Health in Rural Western China" in 2010. This research aimed to effectively arrange health human resources of rural western China under the context of NHCR, by studying on the quality, quantity, distribution, future demands of human health resources, and evaluating factors, policies and management measures that affecting retention and distribution of health workforce. As an outcome of deployment and retention of human health resources, health service quality was analyzed, one appraisal aspect of which was analysis on outpatient prescribing behavior of health institutions, i. e. rational medicine prescribing. The outpatient prescriptions were sampled with randomization from three tiers of health institutions: village healthcare clinics (VHCs), township heath centers (THCs), county-level hospitals (CHs), in the rural areas of 7 provinces (Gansu, Guangxi, Guizhou, Ningxia, Sichuan, Xizang and Xinjiang)[①] of western China in 2012. The planned criteria for selecting the sites of three tiers of health institutions in each province was to select 3 counties based on the discrepancy of economic development (GDP per capita): good, moderate and poor, then to select 3 towns in each county with systematic sampling by ranking the towns with population, and finally to randomly select 3 villages in each town. Commonly, there was only one grassroots health institution in each village and each town, so the VHC and the THC there were certainly selected. To ensure the sample size of the CHs selected into the research, 3 CHs (people's hospital, TCM hospital, and maternal and child health hospital) were chosen in each county. The actual quantity and distribution of three tiers of health institutions is showed in Table 3-2.

Table 3-2   The quantity and the distribution of three tiers of health institutions in the analysis on the status of RUM at the in-depth stage of the NHCR

	No. of VHCs	No. of THCs	No. of CHs
Gansu	15	6	4
Guangxi	19	8	9
Guizhou	8	9	4
Ningxia	11	8	7
Sichuan	24	8	9
Xinjiang	—	9	7
Xizang	—	9	3
Total	77	57	43

3.3.3   Literature and document review

Official documents from international health organizations, such as WHO, INRUD, HAI, DAP and so on, national documents and statistical yearbooks from NHFPC (MoH as former) and NDRC, and provincial

---

①   The whole project was conducted in all the 11 western provinces of China, but the other 4 provinces (Shaanxi, Qinghai, Neimenggu and Yunnan) is not included in this part, so the prescription data for these 4 provinces is not applicable.

documents from local health authorities were reviewed to fully understand the policies context and to obtain supporting data. The peer reviewed papers from domestic and international journals and other gray literatures regarding RUM were also referenced.

3.4 Sampling and data collection

For the pre and post comparative analysis evaluating the effect of the NEMS on RUM, 10 pieces of prescriptions for each day between August 21st and 30th, 2009 and between August 21st and 30th, 2010 from each involved PHI in Zhejiang and Anhui were randomly collected, and 100 outpatient prescriptions for the first half year of 2009, 2010 and 2011 respectively were sampled randomly from each involved PHI in Shandong and Ningxia, so there were 100 prescription samples for each institution each year. The total number of the valid prescriptions in this analysis was 34,339, as showed in Table 3-3.

Table 3-3　　　Number of prescriptions collected for evaluating
the effect of the NEMS on RUM

	No. of PHIs	No. of Prescriptions		
		2009	2010	2011
Zhejiang	99	9,578	9,803	0
Anhui	40	3,943	3,947	0
Shandong	21	1,248	1,246	1,213
Ningxia	16	1,033	1,219	1,109
Total	176	15,802	16,215	2,322

For evaluating the status of RUM in the three tiers of health institutions in rural western China at the in-depth stage of the NHCR, 15 pieces of outpatient prescriptions were randomly extracted with systematic sampling for each month of the year 2012 from each selected health institution, so there were 180 sample prescriptions for each institution. Altogether, 33,611 valid prescriptions were collected (see Table 3-4).

Table 3-4   Number of prescriptions collected for evaluating the status
of RUM at the in-depth stage of the NHCR

	No. of Prescriptions			
	VHCs	THCs	CHs	Total
Gansu	2,889	1,071	727	4,687
Guangxi	3,205	3,294	1,619	8,118
Guizhou	941	1,624	773	3,338
Ningxia	1,825	1,792	1,235	4,852
Sichuan	4,346	1,415	1,543	7,304
Xinjiang	—	1,620	1,260	2,880
Xizang	—	1,620	812	2,432
Total	13,206	12,436	7,969	33,611

3.5   Data processing and analysis

By using Microsoft Office Excel 2010, the prescription data were typed in
and double checked by two individual members of our team, and then coded
and organized for cleaning to ensure there were no errors and omissions.
Missing data were imputed with median value. SPSS 19.0 was applied for
statistical interpretation and statistical inference.

3.5.1   Method used to assess the effect of the NEMS on RUM

Since the onset of the implementation of the NEMS in these sites was in
the year 2010, the year 2009 was considered as prior to the implementation of
the NEMS period, and the year 2010 and the year 2011 were considered as the
post-implementation period.

Based on the SDUIs and referring to the relevant studies, taking the
details extracted from the prescriptions into account, the following six
indicators were used to reflect the change of RUM status between pre- and
post-implementation periods of the NEMS:

(1) Average total number of medicines per prescription;

(2) Average number of EMs per prescription;

(3) Average number of antibiotics per prescription;

(4) Percentage of prescriptions containing antibiotics;

(5) Percentage of prescriptions containing injections;

(6) Percentage of prescriptions containing hormones.

Independent sample t-test and one-way ANOVA were used to compare the mean values of the total number of medicines, the number of EMs and the number of antibiotics for individual prescriptions prior to the implementation of the NEMS with those in the post implementation period. Chi-square test was used to compare the proportions of prescriptions containing antibiotics, injections or hormones before the NEMS implementation with those after the NEMS implementation. If needed, continuity adjustment and Fisher's exact test would be also involved. The results were compared with the standard reference values of RUM for health facilities in developing countries recommended by WHO, if there were any.

3.5.2 Method used to assess the status of RUM at the in-depth stage of NHCR

Apart from those recommended in SDUIs, we also investigated the prescriptions with some more indicators to provide further details of medicine use. The indicators included:

(1) Average total number of medicines per prescription;

(2) Average number of western medicines (WMs) per prescription;

(3) Average number of traditional Chinese medicines (TCMs) per prescription;

(4) Average number of EMs per prescription;

(5) Average number of medicines listed in the medical insurance directories per prescription;

(6) Average number of antibiotics per prescription;

(7) Average number of injections per prescription;

(8) Average number of hormones per prescription;

(9) Percentage of prescriptions containing antibiotics;

(10) Percentage of prescriptions containing injections;

(11) Percentage of prescriptions containing hormones;

(12) Percentage of prescriptions with combined use of antibiotics;

(13) Percentage of prescriptions with combined use of injections;

(14) Average medicine expenses per prescription;

(15) Average proportion of medicine expenses in a prescription.

The indicators (1)-(5) present basic medicine use status, (6)-(13) are the RUM sensitive markers, and (14)-(15) reflect the expense burden of prescribed medicines on patients.

The overall status was assessed as well as the RUM status grouped by provinces and by health institution levels. Descriptive statistics and comparasion means analysis were used to present the results.

3. 5. 3　Method used to establish a comprehensive evaluation index

We used PCA to establish a comprehensive method for evaluating RUM in a health institution. PCA can synthesize original indicators into fewer linearly unrelated principal components that embody the major information of the original indicators by orthogonal transformation. By determining eigenvalues (λ_i) and eigenvectors $[a_i = (a_{i1}, a_{i2}, \cdots, a_{im})', i = 1, 2, \cdots, m]$, principal components ($Z_i = a'\lambda_i X = a_{i1} X_1 + a_{i2} X_2 + \cdots + a_{im} X_m, i = 1, 2, \cdots, m$) is generated. The information contained in the indicators is measured by their variances (λ_i), so PCA is to discompose the total variance of m-original indicators ($X_1, X_2, \cdots, X_m$) into the sum of the variances ($\sum_{i=1}^{m} \lambda_i$) of m-unrelated aggregative indicators ($Z_1, Z_2, \cdots, Z_m$), making the variance of the first principal component (λ_1) the greatest and ranking $\lambda_1, \lambda_2, \cdots, \lambda_m$ from the maximum to the minimum. In general, $\lambda_i / \sum_{i=1}^{m} \lambda_i$ is called the contribution of principal component Z_i and $\sum_{i=1}^{k} (\lambda_i / \sum_{i=1}^{m} \lambda_i)$ is the accumulating contribution of the first k principal components. Not all of the principal components are needed, the criteria for selecting the first k principal components in this study is to keep the present p ($k = p$) principal components when accumulating contribution above 70% or their eigenvalues $\lambda_i \geqslant 1$. The relation between principal components and original indicators can be revealed by factor loading

matrix ($Q = (q_{ij})_{p \times p} = \begin{bmatrix} \sqrt{\lambda_1} a_{11} & \sqrt{\lambda_1} a_{12} & \cdots & \sqrt{\lambda_1} a_{1m} \\ \sqrt{\lambda_2} a_{21} & \sqrt{\lambda_2} a_{22} & \cdots & \sqrt{\lambda_2} a_{2m} \\ \vdots & \vdots & \vdots & \vdots \\ \sqrt{\lambda_m} a_{m1} & \sqrt{\lambda_m} a_{m2} & \cdots & \sqrt{\lambda_m} a_{mm} \end{bmatrix}$). In fact, factor loading (q_{ij}) is the correlation coefficient between principal component Z_i and original indicator X_j, which can disclose the closeness and direction of the relationship. A synthetic evaluation function can be structured by using the selected principal components with contributions as weight ($c_i = \lambda_i / \sum_{i=1}^{m} \lambda_i$): $I = c_1 Z_1 + c_2 Z_2 + \cdots + c_p Z_p$.

To compare the scores and to establish a valid comprehensive evaluation index, the data of original indicators need a transformation at the very beginning to make sure that all the indicators toward the same direction following "a larger score indicating a better outcome" principle to reflect the real situation. (Hoyle, 1973) The approaches to make the inverse original indicators positive we use in this study are: reciprocal method for absolute numbers and 1- method for relative numbers such as percentages. Also, to take Z_i as principal component score, the data of original indicators need to be normalized first. In this research, a 0-1 normalization method is used [$X'_{ij} = (X_{ij} - \overline{X_j})/S_j, j = 1, 2, 3, \cdots, m$].

The original indicators are selected based on those in Section 3.5.2, and the selected ones are the best to reflect the status of RUM:

(1) Average total number of medicines per prescription (X_1);

(2) Average number of EMs per prescription (X_2);

(3) Percentage of prescriptions containing antibiotics (X_3);

(4) Percentage of prescriptions containing injections (X_4);

(5) Percentage of prescriptions containing hormones (X_5);

(6) Average medicine expenses per prescription (X_6);

(7) Average proportion of medicine expenses in a prescription (X_7).

X_1, X_2, X_3 and X_4 are adapted from SDUIs prescription indicators, which scale the performance of rational prescribing. X_5 is chosen to be a supplementary prescription indicator to reflect the hormone use, which is reported to be widely overused in China. X_6 and X_7 are selected to explore the medicine expenditure burden from a patient perspective. X_1 and X_6 are transformed positive with reciprocal method, while X_3, X_4, X_5 and X_7 are transformed positive with 1- method, so that all variables point to the same direction: the larger, the better.

3. 5. 4　Method used to identify the organizational factors that affect the achievement of RUM

The exploratory study on organizational factors that affect the achievement of RUM was built on a conceptual framework and organizational factors that differed from one level of health institutions to another, because the characteristics of different levels of health institutions are quite distinct.

The organizational factors for VHCs are:

(1) Ownership;

(2) Whether to adopt the zero mark-up policy;

(3) Percentage of EMs outfitted.

(4) Number of health workers;

(5) Percentage of financial subsidy from government;

(6) Percentage of revenue from medicines;

(7) Financial subsidy from government per capita;

(8) Revenue from medicines per capita;

The organizational factors for THCs are:

(1) Whether to adopt the SREB;

(2) Number of health workers;

(3) Average number of outpatients per prescriber;

(4) Average number of outpatient prescriptions per prescriber;

(5) Percentage of health workers who received training of the NEMS;

(6) Average income of health workers;

(7) Percentage of financial subsidy from government;

(8) Percentage of revenue from outpatient medicines;

(9) Financial subsidy from government per capita;

(10) Revenue from outpatient medicines per capita.

The organizational factors for CHs are:

(1) Whether to adopt the SREB;

(2) Number of health workers;

(3) Average number of outpatient prescriptions per prescriber;

(4) Average income of health workers;

(5) Percentage of financial subsidy from government;

(6) Percentage of revenue from outpatient medicines;

（7）Financial subsidy from government per capita；

（8）Revenue from outpatient medicines per capita.

These organizational characteristics could be categorized into three groups：institution setting，which reveals institution nature and adoption of related policies；manpower support，such as workload and income of health workers，which may affect the prescribing behaviors；and funding structure and fiscal incentives，which may have an impact on the sustainability of health institutions.

Univariate analysis and multivariate analysis were both employed，with the comprehensive evaluation index I as dependent variable and the organizational characteristics of health institutions as independent variables. The relation between the dependent variable and the independent variables was explored first through the univariate analysis，including t-test，ANOVA， simple linear regression （SLR），etc. to screen meaningful independent variables for multivariate analysis. This was because the sample size was not considerably large，if too many independent variables were involved in multivariate analysis，estimation of model parameters was unstable，affecting model fitting. In order to suppress bias and loss of useful information，the inclusive criteria was set as $p \leqslant 0.30$ accordingly. Multiple linear regression （MLR）models were developed then，with stepwise approach with entry criteria $p \leqslant 0.05$ and removal criteria $p > 0.10$.

Chapter 4 Result I:
The Effect of the NEMS on RUM

4.1 Total medicines prescribed per encounter

The average total number of medicines per prescription is an indicator for the excessive use of medicines. As shown in Table 4-1, compared with the average total number of medicines per prescription for 2009, the indicator for 2010 dropped in every province. In Zhejiang, the richest province of these 4 provinces, this decline was the largest, with a difference of 0.29, and was statistically significant ($p<0.000$), though the other 3 provinces were not. It can also be seen in Table 4-1 that in Shandong and Ningxia, the average total number of medicines per prescription increased from 2010 to 2011.

Table 4-1　　　**Average total number of medicines per prescription**

	2009	2010	2011	DD*	p
Zhejiang	3.56	3.27	—	−0.29	0.000 *
Anhui	4.19	4.05	—	−0.14	0.125
Shandong	3.37	3.28	3.36	−0.01	0.584
Ningxia	3.23	3.12	3.15	−0.08	0.296

* The difference between the values for 2009 and 2010

In comparison with the WHO standard reference value: 1.6-2.8 medicines per outpatient prescription for reasonable prescribing, the mean values of the total number of medicines used per prescription in the PHIs of these 4 provinces were still relatively high even after the NEMS implementation.

4.2 EMs use

The average number of EMs per prescription is an indicator for the use of essential medicines to evaluate the direct effect of the NEMS. According to Table 4-2, compared with the average number of EMs per prescription for 2009, the indicator for the last available year in every province increased, and each difference was statistically significant. In Zhejiang, the difference was the largest, with a value of 0.61. In Shandong, there was a slight drop of the value between 2009 and 2010, but the value went up by 0.6 between 2010 and 2011.

Table 4-2 **Average number of EMs per prescription**

	2009	2010	2011	D*	p
Zhejiang	2.11	2.72	—	0.61	0.000
Anhui	3.13	3.52	—	0.39	0.000
Shandong	1.71	1.62	2.21	0.50	0.000
Ningxia	2.47	2.5	3.01	0.54	0.000

* The difference between the values for 2009 and 2010

The WHO standard reference value for the percentage of EMs in a prescription is 100%. By comparing Table 4-1 and Table 4-2, none of the four provinces reached the standard neither prior to implementation of the NEMS nor in the post implementation period, but the percentage rose after the NEMS implementation in all four provinces.

4.3 Antibiotics use

The average number of antibiotics per prescription is an important indicator for the RUM. Table 4-3 shows that there was a slight fall of the average number of antibiotics per prescription for 2010 in every province compared with that for 2009. The differences in Zhejiang and Ningxia were statistically significant. As can be seen from Table 4-3, there was a fluctuation of the value in Ningxia, and the period from 2009 to 2010 witnessed a remarkable rise in the average number of antibiotics per prescription, which was followed by a relatively sharp decrease between 2010 and 2011. With further independent sample t-test, we found that the difference of the value in Ningxia between 2009 and 2010 as well as that between 2010 and 2011 was statistically significant (p=0.008 and 0.001, respectively), but the difference between 2009 and 2011 was not (p=0.277).

Table 4-3   **Average number of antibiotics per prescription**

	2009	2010	2011	D*	p
Zhejiang	0.8	0.75	—	−0.05	0.000
Anhui	0.93	0.91	—	−0.02	0.198
Shandong	0.73	0.71	0.66	−0.07	0.135
Ningxia	0.72	0.81	0.70	−0.02	0.002

* The difference between the values for 2009 and 2010

The percentage of prescriptions containing antibiotics is a key indicator for RUM. Table 4-4 reveals that in Zhejiang, Anhui, and Shandong, the proportions of prescriptions containing antibiotics decreased from 2009 to 2010 and 2011, and this decline in Zhejiang was statistically significant. In Ningxia, the proportion went up dramatically from 2009 to 2010 and then dropped rapidly from 2010 to 2011, though the proportion in 2011 was higher than that in 2009.

The WHO standard reference value for the percentage of prescriptions containing antibiotics for outpatient is 20.00% to 26.70%. Compared with the standard value, the proportions of prescriptions containing antibiotics investigated from the PHIs of these 4 provinces were twice to triple higher, even after the NEMS implementation.

Table 4-4   **Proportion of prescriptions containing antibiotics**

	Year	Proportion	D*	χ^2	p
Zhejiang	2009	60.89%	−5.62%	62.820	0.000
	2010	55.27%			

Continued

	Year	Proportion	D*	χ^2	p
Anhui	2009	65.04%	−1.59%	1.738	0.187
	2010	63.45%			
Shandong	2009	51.43%	−4.29%	4.883	0.087
	2010	51.43%			
	2011	47.15%			
Ningxia	2009	53.15%	1.14%	13.788	0.001
	2010	60.28%			
	2011	54.29%			

* The difference between the proportions for 2009 and 2010

4.4   Injections use

The percentage of prescriptions containing injections is another key indicator for RUM. Table 4-5 illustrates that in all 4 provinces, the proportions of prescriptions with injections dropped. In Zhejiang, the difference of the proportion was statistically significant, with a decline of 4.14%. In Ningxia, the proportion dropped slightly from 2009 to 2010, and there was a considerable reduction of the proportion between 2010 and 2011.

The WHO standard reference value for the percentage of prescriptions containing injections for outpatient is 13.40% to 24.10%. The proportions of prescriptions containing injections investigated from the PHIs of these 4 provinces are higher than the standard, especially those from Zhejiang and Anhui, except for the proportion of prescriptions from Ningxia after the NEMS implementation.

Table 4-5   Proportion of prescriptions containing injections

	Year	Proportion	DD*	χ^2	p
Zhejiang	2009	44.82%	−4.14%	33.871	0.000
	2010	40.68%			

Continued

	Year	Proportion	DD*	χ^2	p
Anhui	2009	50. 75%	−0. 72%	0. 327	0. 568
	2010	50. 03%			
Shandong	2009	30. 59%	−3. 91%	3. 884	0. 143
	2010	29. 28%			
	2011	26. 68%			
Ningxia	2009	28. 27%	−5. 86%	12. 590	0. 002
	2010	28. 01%			
	2011	22. 40%			

* The difference between the proportions for 2009 and 2010

4. 5   Hormones use

The percentage of prescriptions containing hormones is an indicator that to evaluate the rational use of medicines, since it was reported that the abuse of hormone in China was very common and serious. (Liu & Gao, 2006) As shown in Table 4-6, the proportions of prescriptions containing hormones went down from 2009 to 2010 in Zhejiang and Anhui, with statistical significance. In Shandong and Ningxia, the proportions fluctuated from 2009 to 2011, without statistical significance. In Shandong, the proportion decreased from 2009 to 2010 and then rose between 2010 and 2011, while in Ningxia, the case was the opposite. The proportion containing hormones varied greatly among the 4 provinces, with more than 20% in Anhui and only around 2% in Ningxia.

Table 4-6   Proportion of prescriptions containing hormones

Year	Proportion	DD*	χ^2	p
2009	12. 42%	−2. 88%	41. 206	0. 000
2010	9. 54%			
2009	24. 44%	−3. 43%	10. 581	0. 001

Continued

Year	Proportion	DD*	χ^2	p
2010	21.01%			
2009	11.09%	0.11%	0.153	0.926
2010	10.68%			
2011	11.20%			
2009	1.65%	0.25%	1.257	0.533
2010	2.29%			
2011	1.90%			

* The difference between the proportions for 2009 and 2010

4.6　Discussion

4.6.1　Use of EMs

After the implementation of the NEMS, the quantity of medicines used in a single prescription reduced and the quantity of EMs used increased significantly, so the proportion of EMs used in individual prescription should be raised. It is apparent from the results that the use of EMs in the PHIs of the sample areas was promoted. However, the goal of the policy was to use only EMs in PHIs, which had been already achieved in some other areas in China. (Li et al., 2012) That is to say, the policy effect was not good enough in the sample areas, so that it called for improvement. The reasons for the defect may come to these two points: firstly, it was just the beginning of the NEMS implementation, and the stock of non-EMs needed to consume, and secondly the EML was probably not adequate for the basic demands of medicines in grassroots clinical practice. (Chen, Shi & Guan, 2013; Mao, Zhang & Chen, 2013) The solution for the former is supervision by government, and the solution for the latter is to revise the EML on demand, and there has been already a revised edition of EML released in 2012.

4.6.2　Rational use of antibiotics, injections and hormones

The overall trend for the use of antibiotics, injections and hormones in the PHIs of the sample areas was on the decrease, which was similar to the researches conducted in other areas in China. (Yang et al., 2013) Nevertheless, in one or two provinces involved in our study, the decrease was not significant; instead, the fluctuation was witnessed, or even there was a minor climb.

The risk of many infectious diseases is getting uncontrollable due to the spread of antimicrobial resistance caused by the improper use of antibiotics. (WHO, 2011a) Hormones can take quick effect but may cause intense and long-term detriment to human bodies. Yet, in China, many prescribers considered antibiotics and hormones as specific medications for infections and inflammations regardless of the causations and the types of the symptoms, which may lead to a lot of overuse and misuse of antibiotics and hormones. (Li, Zhang & Wang, 2013; Liu & Gao, 2007) This may suggest that the transmission and update of medicine knowledge to prescribers, especially to those engaging in grassroots clinical practice, are very important.

Injection is an invasive administration of medicines, which increases the risk of ADRs in terms of drug allergy, infections and physiological imbalance including electrolyte imbalance, hypertension, edema, etc. (Hu, Chang & Yuan, 2011) A large number of patients in China believe that injection is the fastest way to cure disease and often ask the practitioners to prescribe injections for them. So it is very important to enhance the professional ethic education for prescribers and general education of medicines use for the masses. In addition, Tang et al. (2013) have proven that the overall effect of government subsidy on the use of injection is positively significant, so it is necessary to provide appropriate financial support to PHIs to cancel prescribers' incentive of making profit.

In addition, according to the current regulations for prescription, such as Procedures for Prescription and Procedures for Clinical Use of Antibiotics, practitioners in violation of provisions under the regulations should be temporarily deprived of prescription privilege. However, this is determined by the health care institutions. If health care institutions acquiesce in practitioners' behavior for the sake of interest, there will be no punishment for inappropriate prescription. Moreover, even if this punishment is given, it is too mild to control practitioners' prescription. Therefore, punitive mechanism has to be improved to enhance the supervision of prescription.

4.6.3 The variations of medicine use among areas with different socio-econo-mic status

Change of medicine use could affect the revenue of PHIs and hence the sustainability and the development, which are associated with practitioners' income and government financial support. In Zhejiang, the richest province of the four sample areas, all changes were positive and statistically significant. It is sure that the policy took obvious effect in this rich province. In view of the change of economic interests involved in the NEMS implementation, we speculated that there might be some relation between the socioeconomic status of an area and the policy effect there. However, the results from the other three areas could not provide clear evidence for this speculation. In Shandong, the second richest province of these four areas as well as one of the richest provinces in China, NEMS failed to give a better performance than in the other two less-developed areas. To verify this relation, further study is required, which should involve multiple economic indicators, including gross domestic product per capita, average income per capita, government revenue, public health expenditure, etc. in each sample area.

4.6.4 Other policies that could affect RUM

There are several other policies that could affect RUM, but to measure the net effect of a policy is very difficult. The policies that could directly affect RUM, for instance, Procedures for Prescription and Procedures for Clinical Use of Antibiotics, which stipulated the medicine use in prescriptions, were not launched in 2009, but were launched in 2004 and 2012 respectively. Therefore, we believe that the results in this study are possibly not disturbed by these policies. Establishing and developing the basic medical insurance system is another one of the five core parts of the NHCR launched in 2009, which may affect medicine use by limiting the scope of reimbursable medicine expenses and the proportion of reimbursement. Nevertheless, the main objective of this policy is to cover more people, and to focus on the change of financing and payment model. The NEMS, one of the key goals of which is RUM, requires that all of the EMs are in the list of reimbursable medicines, and the reimbursement proportion should be higher than non-EMs, which embodies the effect of the basic insurance system on medicine use.

Chapter 5　Result II:
Establishment of a Comprehensive
Evaluation Method for RUM

5. 1　The status of medicine use at the
in-depth stage of the NHCR

On the whole, the average number of medicines per prescription was
3. 61, 2. 57 for WMS and 1. 03 for TCMs on average. The mean of the number
of medicines listed in the national EML or the PEMLs per prescription was
2. 04 and the average number of those listed in the medical insurance
directories per prescription was 2. 32. The RUM sensitive indicators: average
number of antibiotics, injections and hormones per prescription was 0. 70,
0. 74 and 0. 47 respectively; percentage of prescriptions containing antibiotic,
injections or hormones was 53. 94%, 31. 64% and 5. 32% respectively; and
percentage of prescriptions with combined use of antibiotics and injections was
14. 34% and 19. 06% respectively. The average medicine expense per
prescription was 25. 69 CNY and the average proportion of medicine expense in
a prescription was 84. 30%. The indicators which have a reference to the WHO
standard value were much higher.

5. 1. 1　The status of RUM by region

Table 5-1 lists the status of medicine use in the 7 sample provinces with
15 selected indicators.

Table 5-1   **The status of medicine use in the 7 sample provinces**

	Indicators														
	(1)	(2)	(3)	(4)	(5)	(6)	(7)	(8)	(9)	(10)	(11)	(12)	(13)	(14)	(15)
Gansu	4.05	2.40	1.65	2.44	2.45	0.67	1.04	0.03	51.23%	36.23%	3.07%	14.61%	25.15%	27.91	85.05%
Guangxi	3.89	2.86	1.03	2.56	2.86	0.71	0.98	0.11	54.87%	37.26%	11.39%	15.26%	26.92%	23.54	72.54%
Guizhou	3.63	3.12	0.51	2.65	2.67	0.46	1.02	0.05	37.00%	28.04%	5.03%	7.52%	23.34%	45.37	92.39%
Ningxia	2.94	2.26	0.68	2.59	2.81	0.44	0.51	0.02	33.91%	19.49%	1.55%	6.52%	14.26%	18.37	66.13%
Sichuan	4.47	2.37	1.10	2.73	2.68	0.80	0.45	0.05	66.91%	29.63%	5.42%	12.57%	11.08%	20.72	91.25%
Xinjiang	3.72	2.04	1.68	2.75	2.97	1.35	0.69	0.04	77.08%	47.29%	3.51%	43.54%	17.60%	25.79	90.52%
Xizang	2.48	2.18	0.30	2.33	2.34	0.62	0.38	0.02	53.87%	21.26%	2.34%	6.83%	10.70%	21.45	79.77%

Note:

(1) Average total number of medicines per prescription

(2) Average number of WMs per prescription

(3) Average number of TCMs per prescription

(4) Average number of EMs per prescription

(5) Average number of medicines listed in the medical insurance directories per prescription

(6) Average number of antibiotics per prescription

(7) Average number of injections per prescription

(8) Average number of hormones per prescription

(9) Percentage of prescriptions containing antibiotics

(10) Percentage of prescriptions containing injections

(11) Percentage of prescriptions containing hormones

(12) Percentage of prescriptions with combined use of antibiotics

(13) Percentage of prescriptions with combined use of injections

(14) Average medicine expenses per prescription

(15) Average proportion of medicine expenses in a prescription

The average number of medicines per prescription for the provinces (2. 48-4. 47) was much higher than the WHO standard value (1. 6-2. 8), except for the indicator of Xizang, which was in the standard range and was near the upper limit. In 5 out of the 7 provinces, the average quantity of medicines used in a prescription was more than 3. 5; medicines used per encounter in Gansu and Sichuan were more than 4. 0 which were about twice as many as recommended. It also reveals that the quantity of WMs used in a prescription (2. 04-3. 12) accounted for the majority of all medicines, while the usage of TCMs in a prescription (0. 30-1. 68) was much fewer, especially in Xizang (0. 30), Guizhou (0. 51) and Ningxia (0. 68).

The quantities of EMs and the medicines covered by the social medical insurances in a prescription were similar. It also illustrates that the usage of EMs (60. 25%-93. 95%) and medicines covered by the social health insurances (59. 96%-95. 58%) was not concordant with the volume of medicines used in a prescription in most provinces. However, in Ningxia (88. 10% and 95. 58% for the use of EMs and medicines covered by the social health insurances respectively) and Xizang (93. 95% and 94. 35% for the use of EMs and medicines covered by the social health insurances covered respectively), it almost reached the goal of 100% use of EMs as recommended by the standard. In Sichuan, the quantity of EMs in a prescription was greater than the quantity of the medicines listed in the social medical insurance directories, so it could be supposed that some EMs were not covered in any social medical insurance.

The average number of antibiotics, injections and hormones per prescription varied greatly across the provinces. The constituent ratio of antibiotics used in a prescription ranged from 12. 67% to 36. 29%, which was a little greater than that of injections (10. 07%-28. 10%) and even higher than the proportion of hormones (0. 68%-2. 83%). The proportion of prescriptions containing antibiotics was from 33. 91% to 77. 08%. In Xinjiang, this indicator was the highest among the sample provinces, more than twice higher than the lowest Ningxia. Also the prescriptions with combined use of antibiotics accounted for 43. 54% of all prescriptions in Xinjiang, which were much higher than that in other 6 provinces. Unfortunately, even in Ningxia with the lowest proportion of prescriptions containing antibiotics, the indicator was still higher than the WHO standard value (20. 0%-26. 7%). The prescriptions containing injections occupy 47. 29% of all prescriptions in Xinjiang, where the indicator was recorded the highest, while the indicator in Ningxia and Xizang was up to the WHO standard reference value (13. 4%-24. 1%) with 19. 49% and 21. 26% respectively. This indicator was recorded lower than the proportion of the prescriptions containing antibiotics in all the 7 provinces. However, the prescriptions with combined use of injections did not occupy the proportion with prescriptions containing injections, with the highest one of 26. 92% in Guangxi, the median one of 17. 60% in Xinjiang, and the lowest one of 10. 70% in Xizang. The rate of combined use of injections appeared higher than the rate of combined use of antibiotics, except in Sichuan and Xinjiang. The proportion of prescriptions containing hormones was observed ranging from 1. 55% to 11. 39% with the highest in Guangxi, where it was much higher than in any other sample provinces.

The average medicine expense per prescription was RMB 18. 37-45. 37 *yuan*, accounting for 66. 13%-92. 39% of the total expenses. Ningxia was recorded the lowest for both indicators, while Guizhou was recorded the highest.

Overall, the indicators shows that RUM in Ningxia was better than that in any other provinces included in this analysis. In terms of the sensitive indicators, RUM in Xinjiang was the worst, while in terms of the expense of medicines, Guizhou had the heaviest economic burden. Nevertheless, compared with of the WHO standard values, the overall scene was far away from the ideal.

5. 1. 2　The status of RUM by health institution level

Table 5-2 presents the status of RUM across the VHCs, THCs and CHs with 15 selected indicators.

The average total number of medicines per prescription for VHCs, THCs and CHs was 3. 73, 3. 58 and 3. 33 respectively with statistical significance for both ANOVA and multiple comparison ($p = 0.000$). Compared with the WHO standard value (1. 6-2. 8), the parameter values for all the three tiers of health institutions in the rural areas were too high.

The quantity of WMs used in a prescription on average was more than twice than that of TCMs for all the three tiers of health institutions. The deviation of the difference of the number of WMs and TCMs used in a prescription among health institutions of different levels was statistically significant ($F=5073.585$, $p=0.000$). The usage rate of WMs in THCs was the highest (74.30%).

The quantities of EMs used per prescription from VHCs and THCs were the same (2.11), and this for CHs was much lower (1.52) ($F=347.554$, $p=0.000$, and VHCs and THCs in a homogeneous subset while CHs in another by post hoc test with SNK). The usage of EMs was 56.57%, 58.94% and 45.65% of all medicines in a prescription in VHCs, THCs and CHs respectively. The medicines covered by the social medical insurances were used a little more than EMs in a prescription those in VHCs (2.17), while much more than EMs in THCs (2.52) and CHs (2.01). The usage of medicines covered by the social health insurances in a prescription in VHCs, THCs and CHs was 58.18%, 70.39% and 60.36% respectively. In THCs, EMs and medicines covered by the social health insurances were relatively well used, but the usage of EMs was still far from the ideal (100%).

The average number of antibiotics used in a prescription was even higher in THCs (0.83) than in VHCs (0.69) and CHs (0.64) ($F=113.282$, $p=0.000$, and three tiers of health institutions in heterogeneous subsets by SNK test), while the average number of hormones used in a prescription was much lower in THC (0.11) than in VHCs (0.49) and CHs (0.45) ($F=596.691$, $p=0.000$, and three tiers of health institutions in heterogeneous subsets by SNK test). On average, the quantity of injections prescribed per encounter was close between VHCs (0.69) and THCs (0.72) with no statistical significance (in a homogenous subset by SNK test), while the indicator in CHs was somewhat lower (0.62). The percentage of prescriptions containing antibiotics, injections and hormones was 55.70%, 31.41% and 5.89% respectively, of all the prescriptions in THCs, which was a little higher than those in VHCs (54.45%, 28.97%, 4.40%) and in CHs (48.32%, 27.91%, 4.19%) with statistical significance ($p=0.000$, $p=0.025$, $p=0.000$). Compared with the WHO standard values (20.0%-26.7% for antibiotic prescriptions and 13.4%-24.1% for injection prescriptions), the indicators were not good as expected. The prescriptions with combined use of antibiotics

Table 5-2 **The status of medicine use across three tiers of health institutions in the rural areas**

	Indicators														
	(1)	(2)	(3)	(4)	(5)	(6)	(7)	(8)	(9)	(10)	(11)	(12)	(13)	(14)	(15)
VHCs	3.73	2.63	1.10	2.11	2.17	0.69	0.69	0.49	54.45%	28.97%	4.40%	11.72%	20.11%	16.29	80.78%
THCs	3.58	2.66	0.92	2.11	2.52	0.83	0.72	0.11	55.70%	31.41%	5.89%	15.90%	20.22%	23.14	86.88%
CHs	3.33	2.28	1.05	1.52	2.01	0.64	0.62	0.45	48.32%	27.91%	4.19%	14.69%	15.30%	54.84	95.55%

Note:

(1) Average total number of medicines per prescription

(2) Average number of WMs per prescription

(3) Average number of TCMs per prescription

(4) Average number of EMs per prescription

(5) Average number of medicines listed in the medical insurance directories per prescription

(6) Average number of antibiotics per prescription

(7) Average number of injections per prescription

(8) Average number of hormones per prescription

(9) Percentage of prescriptions containing antibiotics

(10) Percentage of prescriptions containing injections

(11) Percentage of prescriptions containing hormones

(12) Percentage of prescriptions with combined use of antibiotics

(13) Percentage of prescriptions with combined use of injections

(14) Average medicine expenses per prescription

(15) Average proportion of medicine expenses in a prescription

and those with combined use of injections went the similar way as independent use, accounting for 15. 90% and 20. 22% respectively, of all the prescriptions in THCs, a little higher than those in VHCs and CHs with statistical significance ($p=0.000$, $p=0.012$).

The average medicine expense and the average proportion of medicine cost in a prescription rose with the elevation of the health institution level ($F=4.426$, $p=0.000$, and $F=3.514$, $p=0.000$, in both mean comparison, three tiers of health institutions in heterogeneous subsets by post hoc SNK test). In CHs, the average medicine expense per prescription (54. 84 *yuan*) was much higher than those in THCs (23. 14 *yuan*) and in VHCs (16. 29 *yuan*), so was the average proportion of medicine cost in a prescription, which reached 95. 55%.

Overall, the sensitive indicators reveals that RUM in THCs was the worst among the three tiers of health institutions in the rural areas, while the burden of medicines on people in CHs was the heaviest.

5. 2　Establishment of a comprehensive evaluation model

5. 2. 1　Procedure and model parameters

This part presents the process of PCA to constitute a synthetic evaluation function for measuring RUM status by using the prescription data from the three tiers of health institutions in rural western China at the in-depth stage of the NHCR.

The indicators X_1-X_7 presented in this part have been already transformed toward the same direction and performed normalized treatment. Z_i is for the principal components, c_i is for the contribution of factors and I is for the synthetic evaluation value.

Table 5-3 is the matrix for correlation coefficient and significance level. Kaiser-Meyer-Olkin (KMO) test shows that measure of sampling adequacy is 0. 578, which is evaluated miserable by Kaiser and Rice (1974), and Bartlett's test of sphericity derives approximate chi-square of 148. 108 with significance 0. 000, so it is just tolerable to conduct a factor analysis.

Table 5-3   **Correlation matrix**

		X_1	X_2	X_3	X_4	X_5	X_6	X_7
Correlation								
	X_1	1.000	−0.201	0.281	0.101	0.169	0.070	0.031
	X_2	−0.201	1.000	−0.350	−0.199	−0.293	−0.060	0.092
	X_3	0.281	−0.350	1.000	0.487	0.235	0.008	0.064
	X_4	0.101	−0.199	0.487	1.000	0.240	0.030	−0.098
	X_5	0.169	−0.293	0.235	0.240	1.000	−0.050	−0.088
	X_6	0.070	−0.060	0.008	0.030	−0.050	1.000	0.362
	X_7	0.031	0.092	0.064	−0.098	−0.088	0.362	1.000
Sig.(1-tailed)								
	X_1		0.004	0.000	0.091	0.012	0.178	0.339
	X_2	0.004		0.000	0.004	0.000	0.214	0.113
	X_3	0.000	0.000		0.000	0.001	0.458	0.198
	X_4	0.091	0.004	0.000		0.001	0.347	0.097
	X_5	0.012	0.000	0.001	0.001		0.253	0.121
	X_6	0.178	0.214	0.458	0.347	0.253		0.000
	X_7	0.339	0.113	0.198	0.097	0.121	0.000	

Table 5-4 illustrates how much variance is explained by the components. The first two components have an eigenvalue ($\geqslant 1$), about 10% of the variance was discovered in the fifth factor, and the first four components accounted for 74.425% of the total variance. Therefore, the first four factors are kept as principal components. Figure 5-1 presents the decline of eigenvalues and accumulative variance contribution rate. After Z_3, the eigenvalues are less than 1, and the broken line becomes gentle.

Table 5-4   **Total variance explained**

Component	Eigenvalues		
	Total	Variance (%)	Cumulative (%)
Z_1	2.058	29.400	29.400

Continued

Component	Eigenvalues		
	Total	Variance (%)	Cumulative (%)
Z_2	1.397	19.956	49.356
Z_3	0.923	13.184	62.540
Z_4	0.832	11.884	74.425
Z_5	0.731	10.444	84.869
Z_6	0.662	9.451	94.320
Z_7	0.398	5.680	100.000

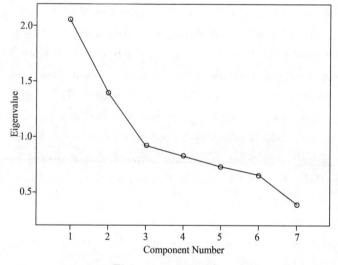

Figure 5-1　Scree Plot

Table 5-5 reflects the relationship between components (Z_i) and original indicators (X_i). The entries of the matrix are called factor loadings, which are actually the coefficients of correlation that provide the extent of close relation and the effect direction.

Table 5-5　　　　　　　　**Factor loading matrix**

	Z_1	Z_2	Z_3	Z_4
X_1	0.486	0.201	−0.600	0.550
X_2	−0.648	0.011	0.273	0.377

Continued

X_3	0.776	0.119	0.264	0.262
X_4	0.668	-0.052	0.601	0.097
X_5	0.587	-0.167	-0.226	-0.478
X_6	0.033	0.801	0.029	-0.283
X_7	-0.094	0.819	0.068	0.008

The factor loading matrix indicates that the first principal component (Z_1) explains the use of antibiotics, injections and EMs (negative) (X_2, X_3 and X_4) loading explicitly high (>0.6), with total amount of medicines used and the use of hormones (X_1 and X_5) loads relatively high (>0.4); the second principal component (Z_2) associated with medicine expenditure and its proportion out of total cost in a prescription (X_6 and X_7) explicitly loads very high (>0.8); the third principal component (Z_3) is correlative to total medicine use in a prescription (negative) and the use of injections (X_1 and X_4) explicitly loads high (>0.6); and the fourth principal component (Z_4) connected with total amount of medicines used and the use of hormones (negative) (X_1 and X_5) loads high (>0.4). In general, Z_1 can draw a fairly comprehensive picture for the medicine use and Z_2 can strongly reflect the medicine burden. On account of the cumulative contribution of Z_1 and Z_2 is too low, we retain Z_3 and Z_4, which provide partial information about the medicine use, in the model.

According to these factor loadings, the principal components are calculated as:

$Z_1 = 0.339X_1 - 0.451X_2 + 0.541X_3 + 0.466X_4 + 0.409X_5 + 0.023X_6 - 0.066X_7$;

$Z_2 = 0.170X_1 + 0.009X_2 + 0.101X_3 - 0.044X_4 - 0.141X_5 + 0.678X_6 + 0.693X_7$;

$Z_3 = -0.625X_1 + 0.284X_2 + 0.275X_3 + 0.626X_4 - 0.235X_5 + 0.030X_6 + 0.071X_7$;

$Z_4 = 0.604X_1 + 0.414X_2 + 0.287X_3 + 0.106X_4 - 0.524X_5 - 0.311X_6 + 0.009X_7$.

Then the synthetic appraisal function is generated as:

$I = 0.294Z_1 + 0.19956Z_2 + 0.13184Z_3 + 0.11884Z_4$.

The capitalized I means the better RUM status.

5.2.2 Model validation

Model validation was used as a comprehensive evaluation index to assess RUM in the sample health institutions, and compare its values with the results in Section 5.1.

The mean of I for the 177 sample health institutions was 0.0000, of course, with 95% confidence interval $(-0.0758, 0.0758)$ and standard error 0.3842. The median of I was 0.0289, higher than the mean, indicating that RUM in some institutions was much worse than the average. The minimum I was -1.18 and the the maximum was 1.54, and the standard deviation (SD) was 0.5112.

Table 5-6 presents the values of the four principal components and the comprehensive evaluation index for RUM in the sample health institutions. Ningxia achieved the highest I score with the highest values of Z_1 and Z_2, which means that in both terms of medicine use condition and medicine expense burden, the RUM status in Ningxia was better than those in other sample regions. Sichuan got the lowest Z_1, Guizhou and Xinjiang received the lowest Z_2, and the lowest I score went for Xinjiang, representing the worst RUM status among the sample provinces. The difference of I scores among provinces has statistical significance ($p = 0.000$). These approximately tally with the results given by Table 5-1. Figure 5-2 shows I score distribution of the health institutions by regions.

Table 5-6   **RUM comprehensive evaluation scores by regions**

	No. of Health Institutions	Z_1	Z_2	Z_3	Z_4	I
Gansu	25	-0.3345	-0.2660	0.1013	-0.0078	-0.1390
Guangxi	36	-0.4986	0.4902	0.3812	0.2700	0.0940
Guizhou	21	1.1059	-0.4910	0.0094	-0.4481	0.1951
Ningxia	26	1.3682	0.7929	-0.5930	0.8446	0.5223
Sichuan	41	-0.7859	-0.3216	0.2798	-0.1573	-0.2770
Xinjiang	16	-0.3475	-0.5149	-0.8859	-1.0408	-0.4454
Xizang	12	0.4413	0.4170	0.1390	0.0858	0.0750

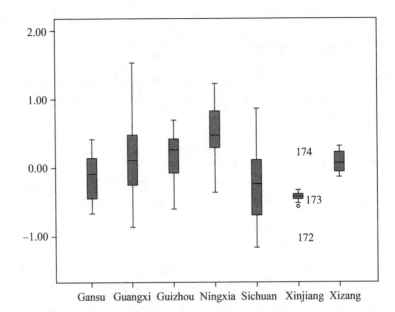

Figure 5-2　Box Plot for I Scores by Province

According to Table 5-7, VHCs scored the highest I while THCs got the lowest, indicating that VHCs had a better RUM condition while THCs had a relatively worse condition. The score of Z_2, which reflects the medicine burden, for CHs was the lowest. The difference of I scores among organizations has statistical significance ($p = 0.007$). These agree with the findings shown in Table 5-1. Figure 5-3 presents I score distribution of the health institutions by institutions.

Table 5-7　　RUM comprehensive evaluation scores by health institutions

	No. of Health Institutions	Z_1	Z_2	Z_3	Z_4	I
VHCs	77	−0.1340	0.4144	0.0090	−0.0954	0.0332
THCs	57	−0.1503	−0.0460	0.0635	0.1059	−0.0324
CHs	43	0.4392	−0.6812	−0.1003	0.0304	−0.0164

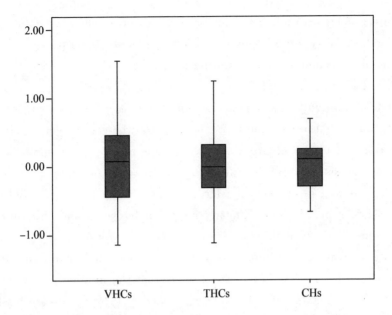

Figure 5-3   Box Plot for *I* Scores by Health Institutions

By comparing the comprehensive evaluation scores for RUM with the descriptive results, it can be regarded that the model is adequate and effective.

5. 3   Discussion

5. 3. 1   Unsatisfactory RUM status at the in-depth stage of the NHCR

Taking the WHO recommended reference values for SDUIs as criterion, almost every indicator derived from the data in outpatient prescriptions from the health institutions across every sample region or every organizational level was unsatisfactory. Excess use of medicines remained prevalent, and improper polypharmacy and use of antibiotics and injections was the main impediment to RUM achievement. Xiao et al. (2016) presented similar results in their published paper, indicating that inappropriate antibiotic use was a serious problem in primary health institutions in China even if the NEMS had been enforced. Moreover, the percentage of EMs prescribed in an outpatient prescription was not high enough, leaving much space for non-EMs. Meanwhile, medicine expense and its proportion in total cost of a prescription kept high, along with under-use of social health insurance covered medicines. Hence affordability of medicines in the outpatient prescriptions was low, bringing about economic burden on the patients.

A large discrepancy of RUM status among different regions seems not tightly bound up with the development of economics. This is similar to what has been discussed in Chapter 4. We believe that the causes were complicated and various, and conjecture that there were plenty of reasons, such as prevalence of disease, fulfillment of policy, natural environment and social condition, as well as economics. Mardan et al. (2014) find that utilization of health services in THCs in Xinjiang increased by years and the number of surgical operations was above the national average. More operations brought about the increase of antibiotics use, rise of prescription charge and indirect reduction of EMs use. We find in our study that the number of prescriptions with operation related diagnosis, e. g. congenital heart disease (CHD), pancreatectomy, cerebral infarction, stroke, appendicitis and tumors, in Xinjiang was higher than that in any other regions. This could somewhat explain the severe RUM status in Xinjiang . Also in Xinjiang, a study shows that there was a lack of confidence in the compensation mechanism after the implementation of the NEMS among a considerable quantity of health institutions in rural areas. (Li et al., 2015) SREB had not been carried out yet due to sophisticated capital composition of the health institutions. In Xizang, a vast high-altitude territory with a sparse population, cold and dry climate, and relative sealing environment, drug-resistant strain was less than that in other regions and pathogenic bacteria was high sensitive to medicines, so the consumption of antibiotics was much though the variety was single. Meanwhile, Xizang was less developed and short of health services, and medicines in health institutions in rural areas were sourced from allotment and donation of government and army. Therefore, there was less usage of medicines and combined medications, and prescription cost was lower.

RUM status differed in different levels of health institutions. THCs appeared the worst. Wan et al. (2014) believes that EMs outfitted in THCs were not sufficient and unable to satisfy the clinical medication needs, because EML was not perfect, and dispatch and delivery of EMs were inefficient. They also considers that the health staff allocation was inappropriate in THCs, with shortage of health personnel, aged experienced workers, few new members, and difficulty in attracting and retaining high educated talents because of finite funding. It was supposed that SREB without an adequate reimbursement mechanism could not eliminate the motivation of making profits from drugs by overprescribing medicines, especially antibiotics and injections. The high medicine expense in the prescriptions from CHs should be attributed to the following reasons: (1) CHs, as centers for health services and medical techniques of a county, took on diagnosis and treatment of common and frequently-encountered diseases as well as some special medical services, e.g. rescuing of critical diseases and diagnosis and treatment of difficult miscellaneous diseases for people in rural areas, so that the business was complex and use of medicines was diverse and in large quantities, and also a lot of non-EMs should be used; (2) Comprehensive reform of CHs with implementation of the zero mark-up policy for EMs was just launched then, requiring time to fulfill the policy goals.

5.3.2 Appropriateness and deficiency of the comprehensive evaluation method and its establishment

5.3.2.1 PCA versus factor analysis

PCA is a widely used technique for dimension reduction to extract main features of original variables, which is closely related to factor analysis. PCA and factor analysis can be both geared to exploratory factor analysis (EFA), which is used to spot sophisticated interrelationships among items that are part of consolidated concepts with no priori assumptions about relationships. PCA is the first phase of EFA. Fabrigar et al. (1999) presents a number of reasons suggesting they are not identical. PCA transforms multiple indicators into fewer synthetic indicators that are called principal components containing as much information of original variables as possible and with no mutuality among one another. Factor analysis describes variability among observed, correlated variables in terms of a potentially lower number of unobserved variables called factors, which represent the common variance of variables, with minimum loss of information. Moreover, KMO test is required when conducting factor analysis, with value ≥ 0.7 for appropriateness and value < 0.5 for abandonment, while PCA is not required for this since its result is determined by data structure. In our study, KMO measure of sampling adequacy was 0.578, and this is miserable for factor analysis. Furthermore, PCA can derive individual scores for components and a composite score to overall evaluation, while such information cannot be yielded from factor analysis. Therefore, PCA is selected in this study to synthetically evaluate the RUM status with I score.

5.3.2.2　Principal components selection

Only Z_1 and Z_2's eigenvalues λ_1, λ_2 are greater than 1 and these two principal components could represent RUM sensitive indicators and medicine expense indicators respectively. However, their accumulative contribution is too small, less than 50%, indicating that there may be a great loss of information if we just keep these two principal components. Therefore, Z_3 and Z_4 are also enclosed in the model as supplementary explanations for medicine use to make the accumulative contribution more than 70%.

It is generally believed that eigenvalues λ_i should not be less than 1, or it means that the explanatory ability of the principal components is weaker than the original indicators. This may be due to the high correlativity among the original indicators, suggesting that there exist some viable alternatives for selecting indicators that reflect RUM status. Actually, the principal components Z_1 and Z_2 could preferably reflect the most important two sectors of RUM: medicine dosage and medicine expense. However, since we planned to establish an aggregative indicator I for evaluating RUM, as much information as possible was retained in the function. And the results of original indicators and comprehensive index appear similar in our study, indicating the validity of the model is still good.

Chapter 6　Result III:
Organizational Barriers Associated with
the Achievement of RUM

6. 1　Organizational barriers associated with the achievement of RUM in VHCs

For VHCs, the following organizational indicators were explored through univariate analysis and multivariate analysis: ownership; whether to adopt the zero mark-up policy; percentage of EMs outfitted; number of health workers; percentage of financial subsidy from government; percentage of revenue from medicines; financial subsidy from government per capita; and revenue from medicines per capita.

The majority of the VHCs were village-run (44. 16%) or town-run (25. 97%), and town-run VHCs obtained much higher I than VHCs of any other patterns of ownership (see Table 6-1). One-way ANOVA for identifying the relation between RUM score I and ownership was performed ($F=2.552$, $p=0.035$).

Table 6-1　　　　　　　　　**Ownership of the VHCs**

Ownership	Frequency	Percentage	Mean of I
Village-Run	34	44. 16	−0. 0695
Town-Run	20	25. 97	0. 4170
Joint	9	11. 69	−0. 1449
Private	9	11. 69	−0. 1509
Other	5	6. 49	−0. 1528

70 VHCs adopted the zero mark-up policy while another 7 did not (see Table 6-2). The difference of I scores between the two groups was not statistically significant ($p=0.801$).

Table 6-2   **Zero mark-up policy adoption of the VHCs**

Zero Mark-up Policy Adoption	Frequency	Percentage	Mean of I
Adopted	70	90.91	0.0276
Not Adopted	7	9.09	0.0888

The percentage of EMs outfitted in the VHCs was 90.65% on average. 42 VHCs achieved the goal of 100% outfitted medicines, while some VHC outfitted EMs accounting for only 24.01% of all medicines provided. Simple linear regression (SLR) of RUM score I on percentage of EMs failed, as F test resulted in no significance ($\beta=0.368$, $p=0.419$).

Most of the VHCs only had no more than 3 health workers (77.92%), while the number of health workers at most in the VHCs was 11 (Table 6-3). One-way ANOVA of SLR showed that the relation between RUM score I and number of health workers was not statistically significant ($\beta=-0.055$, $p=0.132$).

Table 6-3   **Number of health workers in the VHCs**

No. of Health Workers	Frequency	Percentage (%)	Mean of I
1	20	25.97	-0.0388
2	23	29.87	0.2867
3	17	22.08	-0.1854
4	8	10.39	0.0745
$\geqslant 5$	9	11.69	-0.0185

Averagely, 28.23% of the income of the VHCs was from governmental financial subsidy. In some VHCs, the subsidy held 86.60% of the revenue, while there were 6 VHCs receiving no financial subsidy at all. However, the average proportion of medicines revenue was 52.37%, with a minimum of 23.60% and a maximum of 88.75%. SLR results reveal the significance of the correlation between RUM score I and revenue structure, with $p=0.059$ and $\beta=0.551$ for proportion of governmental financial subsidy and $p=0.021$ and $\beta=-0.685$ for proportion of medicine revenues, respectively.

The mean of governmental financial subsidy per health worker was RMB 5,424.31 *yuan* in these VHCs, one of which obtained the most subsidy per capita of RMB 57,200 *yuan*, while medicines revenue per capita was RMB 12,886.23 *yuan* on average, varying greatly with a minimum of RMB 181.82 *yuan* and a maximum of RMB 70,000 *yuan*. The correlations between RUM score I and VHCs' revenues per capita were not statistically significant with $p=0.190$ and $\beta=1.197 \times 10^{-5}$ for financial subsidy from government per capita and $P=0.969$ and $\beta=-1.996 \times 10^{-7}$ for revenue from prescribing medicines per capita.

Accordingly, ownership, number of health workers, percentage of financial subsidy from government, percentage of revenue from medicines and governmental financial subsidy per capita were regarded as meaningful independent variables for multiple linear regression (MLR). Ownership was disposed to dummy variables. Eventually, ownership (town-run) and number of health workers entered into the MLR model, with coefficients of 0.651 ($p=0.000$) and -0.077 ($p=0.022$), respectively. The constant was 0.002. ANOVA for regression on residual indicated the linear relation was established ($p=0.000$). The tolerance was 0.979, i.e. variance inflation factor (VIF) was 1.022, revealing there was no multicollinearity. The coefficient of determination $R^2=0.519$, indicating an acceptable model fitting.

Therefore, town-run VHCs seemed to have a better RUM status, while a large number of health workers had a negative effect on RUM achievement.

6.2 Organizational barriers associated with the achievement of RUM in THCs

For THCs, the following organizational indicators were explored through univariate analysis and multivariate analysis: whether to adopt SREB; number of health workers; average number of outpatients per prescriber; average number of outpatient prescriptions per prescriber; percentage of health workers who received training of the NEMS; average income of health workers; percentage of financial subsidy from government; percentage of revenue from outpatient medicines; financial subsidy from government per capita; and revenue from outpatient medicines per capita.

40 THCs (70.18%) adopted SREB while the other 17 did not (Table 6-4). The difference of I scores between the two groups was not statistically significant ($p = 0.119$).

Table 6-4　　　　　　　SREB adoption of the THCs

Adoption of SREB	Frequency	Percentage	Mean of I
Adopted	40	70.18	-0.1756
Not Adopted	17	29.82	0.0284

The number of health workers in individual THC was 30 on average (Table 6-5). The correlation between RUM score I and number of health workers was not statistically significant ($\beta = -0.003$, $p = 0.162$) in the THCs.

Table 6-5　　　　　Number of health workers in the THCs

No. of Health Workers	Frequency	Percentage	Mean of I
0-19	22	38.60	0.1255
20-39	18	31.58	-0.0202
40-59	12	21.05	-0.3584
$\geqslant 60$	5	8.77	-0.2224

In the THCs, a prescriber saw 1,167 patients (with a minimum of 154 and a maximum of 5,673) and made 1,182 outpatient prescriptions (with a minimum of 116 and a maximum of 6,057) within one year on average. That means in most outpatient encounters, only one Rx was prescribed. The correlation between RUM score I and average number of outpatients per prescriber as well as between RUM score I and average number of outpatient prescriptions per prescriber was not statistically significant, with $p = 0.299$ ($\beta = 5.844 \times 10^{-5}$) and $p = 0.265$ ($\beta = 6.118 \times 10^{-5}$), respectively.

Averagely, about half of the health workers (48.30%) in the THCs received training of the NEMS. However, in some THCs the proportion was only 9.84%, while in some others almost every health worker (98.48%) was well trained of EMs or RUM related policies. The impact of the NEMS training on RUM was not statistically significant ($\beta=0.196$, $p=0.109$).

The mean of health workers' annual income in the THCs was RMB 2,709.65 $yuan$, with a least of RMB 1,700 $yuan$ and a most of RMB 5,553 $yuan$ (SD$=763.062$). SLR showed no statistical significance of the correlation between RUM score I and income of health workers ($\beta=\times10^{-5}$, $p=0.345$).

On average, governmental financial subsidy held more or less half (50.69%) of the THCs' revenue. This proportion varied widely from 11.59% to 88.93%. Also, 14.81% of the earning was from outpatient medicines averagely, with a minimum of 4.29% and a maximum of 38.81%. Another 10.88% of income went for inpatient medications. No statistical significance was found for the correlation between RUM score I and revenue structure ($p=0.305$ and $\beta=0.283$ for percentage of governmental financial subsidy, and $p=0.350$ and $\beta=-0.737$ for percentage of outpatient medicine income).

In these THCs, the mean of governmental financial subsidy per health worker was RMB 53,237 $yuan$, and the most subsidy per capita obtained was RMB 250,000 $yuan$, while medicines revenue per capita was RMB 16,213 $yuan$ on average, differing greatly with a minimum of RMB 3,200 $yuan$ and a maximum of RMB 83,300 $yuan$. The correlations between RUM score I and THCs' revenues per capita were not statistically significant with $p=0.694$ and $\beta=0.006$ for governmental financial subsidy per capita and $p=0.676$ and $\beta=-0.018$ for medicines revenue per capita.

Through univariate analysis, all organizational indicators were detected seemingly of no statistical significance associated with RUM. Since it was an exploratory study, those with $p\leqslant0.3$ were deemed to be meaningful and would be also screened by MLR. They were whether to adopt SREB, number of health workers, average number of outpatients per prescriber, average number of outpatient prescriptions per prescriber, and percentage of health workers who received training of the NEMS. Ultimately, whether to adopt SREB, number of health workers and percentage of health workers who received training of the NEMS were entered into the MLR model, with regression coefficients of -0.133 ($p=0.013$), -0.008 ($p=0.007$) and 0.160 ($p=0.018$), respectively. The constant was 0.201. ANOVA for regression on residual indicated the linear relation was established ($p=0.025$). VIFs were all less than 2 (1.610, 1.570 and 1.062 respectively), revealing there was no multicollinearity. The coefficient of determination R^2 was 0.494, indicating an acceptable model fitting.

Hence, relative abundance of health workers receiving training of the NEMS had a positive impact on RUM, while adopting SREB and a relatively large number of health workers might cause irrational use of medicines in the THCs.

6.3 Organizational barriers associated with the achievement of RUM in CHs

For CHs, the following organizational indicators were explored through univariate analysis and multivariate analysis: whether to adopt SREB, number of health workers, average number of outpatient prescriptions per prescriber, average income of health workers, percentage of financial subsidy from government, percentage of revenue from outpatient medicines, financial subsidy from government per capita, and revenue from outpatient medicines per capita.

The CIIs that adopted SREB were slightly less than those that not adopted (see Table 6-6). The difference of I scores between the two groups was statistically significant ($p=0.000$).

Table 6-6   **SREB adoption of the CHs**

Adoption of SREB	Frequency	Percentage	Mean of I
Adopted	20	46.51	-0.2496
Not Adopted	23	53.49	0.1863

The number of health workers in individual CHs was 205 on average, and about two thirds of the CHs had less than 200 health workers (see Table 6-7). The correlation between RUM score I and number of health workers was not statistically significant ($\beta=0.000$, $p=0.511$) in the CHs.

Table 6-7	Number of health workers in the CHs		
No. of Health Workers	Frequency	Percentage	Mean of I
0-199	28	65. 12	−0. 0595
200-399	7	16. 28	0. 1137
⩾400	8	18. 60	0. 0067

A prescriber in the CHs wrote out an average of 657 outpatient prescriptions within a single year (with a minimum of 52 and a maximum of 1,761). There is no statistical significance of the correlation between RUM score I and the average number of outpatient prescriptions per prescriber in the CHs ($\beta=9.138\times10^{-5}$, $p=0.585$).

The average yearly income of health workers was RMB 3,726.98 *yuan*, with a least of RMB 1,756 *yuan* and a most of RMB 6,663 *yuan* SD = 1,254.093) in the CHs. SLR presented no statistical significance of the correlation between RUM score I and the annual income of health workers ($\beta=8.034\times10^{-5}$, $p=0.101$).

Averagely, governmental financial subsidy held 26.03% of the CHs' total revenue, while outpatient medicines earning occupied 13.22%. Statistical significance was found of the correlation between RUM score I and proportion of governmental financial subsidy ($\beta=-0.557$, $p=0.023$), but the correlation between RUM score I and percentage of outpatient medicines income was not statistically significant ($\beta=0.261$, $p=0.782$).

In these CHs, the mean of governmental financial subsidy per health worker was RMB 54,042 *yuan*, and the least and the most subsidy per capita obtained was RMB 6,957 *yuan* and RMB 435,700 *yuan*, respectively. Medicines revenue per capita was RMB 31,136 *yuan* on average, with a great range between RMB 1,300 *yuan* and RMB 160,400 *yuan*. The correlations between RUM score I and CHs' revenues per capita were not statistically significant with $p=0.196$ and $\beta=-0.009$ for governmental financial subsidy per capita and $p=0.508$ and $\beta=-0.014$ for medicines revenue per capita.

Accordingly, whether to adopt SREB, annual income of health workers, percentage of financial subsidy from government and governmental financial subsidy per health worker were screened as meaningful variables and brought into multivariate analysis. Finally, whether to adopt SREB was entered into the MLR model, with the regression coefficient of -0.385 ($p=0.001$), and the constant was 0.144. ANOVA for regression on residual indicated the linear relation was established ($p=0.001$). The coefficient of determination R^2 was 0.513, indicating an acceptable model fitting.

Thus, not adopting SREB had a positive impact on RUM status in the CHs. This was similar to that in the THCs.

6.4　Discussion

6.4.1　Organizational characteristics differ among different tiers of VHCs, health institutions

The most grass-root health institutions in the three-tier network of disease prevention and healthcare for rural areas, are at the first line and the first place of PHCs. Usually, they are very small with only a couple of medical technicians and a few funding, focusing on public health as well as prevention and healthcare for the local village residents, and their operation is guided by THCs. THCs are the kernel of the rural three-tier network of health service, engaging in medical care and epidemic prevention of the most elementary administrative division of the rural areas where they locate. They are also the sites where NEMS was initiated. However, THCs struggle to maintain operation against VHCs and CHs, because addressing an ailment is more convenient in VHCs, though CHs are much more professional in treating serious diseases. (Zhang, Li & Chen, 2011) CHs are leaders of the three-tier healthcare network in rural areas, treating common and frequently-occurring clinical illness as well as difficult and miscellaneous maladies, saving patients in emergency and critical medical conditions, and providing VHCs and THCs with technical guidance and training. With the public hospital reform, NEMS related policies, e.g. zero mark-up policy, were extended to CHs. CHs are required to meet a majority of health demand of rural population, but are short of professional health workers, necessary medical instrument and sufficient financial funding. The rural three-tier health service network endows distinct functions to VHCs, THCs and CHs, so organizational characteristics of them differ greatly.

Since the data for this study were second hand, some useful variables might not be collected. However, plenty of meaningful cases were discovered still.

With respect to ownership, THCs and CHs in the rural three-tier health service network were public, of which county health bureaus were in charge, while there was a variety of VHCs' ownership due to the lapsed rural cooperative medical systems with self-support village doctors providing healthcare for the village residents, most of which were THC-run or village-committee-run while some remained private and some others were in joint mode.

As for policy adoption, whether to adopt zero mark-up policy and EMs outfit status could reflect the NEMS compliance of the VHCs. The results show that general situation was good but far from perfection, and in some VHCs the situation was much worse than others. SREB was the management syste which aimed to eliminate the motivation of pursuing profit but ensured the sustainability of operation of THCs and CHs. This policy was adopted in approximately 70% of the THCs and around 50% of the CHs.

In accordance with the tier, the VHCs only had a couple of medical staff, the THCs had got scores of health workers, and the CHs gathered hundreds of skillful doctors . Health workers in the THCs took on about twice workload than those in the CHs but got 30% less income. This imparity might compromise the medical service quality, bringing about disharmony and irrational medicines use. In addition, less than half of the health workers in the THCs were well trained of NEMS and RUM. In that the NEMS was projected much on medicines use in PHIs, especially in THCs, health workers' poor knowledge of medicine policies and medicines use might result in policy ineffectiveness.

Table 6-8 summarizes the revenue structure in terms of financial subsidy from government and income from outpatient medicines of the three-tier health institutions. More than half of the revenue in VHCs was from outpatient medicines, while THCs relied much more on governmental financial subsidy to sustain its operation. CHs were complex hospitals, and their revenue composition was much more sophisticated, e.g. hospitalization charge and examination fee, so governmental financial subsidy and outpatient medicines income held no more than 40%. The THCs and the CHs received very similar amounts of governmental subsidy per capita, while VHCs had got much less. The earning from outpatient medicines per capita in CHs was as almost twice as that in the THCs and two and a half times as that in the VHCs.

Table 6-8   Revenue structure of the three-tier health institutions

	Percentage of Governmental Financial Subsidy	Percentage of Outpatient Medicines Revenue	Governmental Financial Subsidy per Health worker (*yuan*)	Outpatient Medicines Revenue per Health Worker (*yuan*)
VHCs	28. 23	52. 37	5,424	12,886
THCs	50. 69	14. 81	53,237	16,213
CHs	26. 03	13. 22	54,042	31,136

6. 4. 2   Organizational barriers associated with the RUM achievement in rural three-tier healthcare network

The organizational barriers associated with the RUM achievement also differed among different tiers of health institutions in rural areas. Firstly, the RUM status in town-run VHCs was evidently better than that in the VHCs with other ownership. Immediate leadership and close operation guidance by THCs brought those VHCs better knowledge of medicines use and better compliance with related polices to promote RUM. Secondly, there was a shortage of high-educated healthcare talents in PHIs, and staff were aged and deficient in working enthusiasm. (Feng et al., 2012) It was possible that health workers overstaffing in the VHCs and THCs brought about low efficiency and irrational use of medicines. Thirdly, it has been verified in the THCs that the more health workers received relevant training, the better the RUM status was. Last but not least, adopting SREB could not lead to reaching the policy goal; instead, it did adverse impact on the RUM achievement in the THCs and the CHs. Zou (2015) believes that this policy required powerful fiscal capacity of a local government, and if the government could not afford the budget, the appropriation would influence the operation of health institutions. This policy also conflicted with the prospective payment system of social medical insurance, reducing the capacity of autonomous operation of a health institution, suppressing the positivity of providing adequate health services, and lowering the pay of the health workers.

This study is an exploratory research, so organizational indicators associated with RUM should be fully determined. In our MLR models, R^2s were around moderate 0.5, and this was advisable because we would not use the models for prediction. Yet, this could also indicate that there might be something meaningful that were not included. It was nice to take more consideration on the organizational indicators with $p > 0.05$ for respective partial regression coefficients in MLR, instead of simply dropping them.

Perverse financial incentive has been always supposed to be a cause of irrational use of medicines. (Reynolds & McKee, 2009) In this study, relatively high remuneration of health workers could seemingly improve prescribing pattern as well. However, some researchers pointed out that the removal of pecuniary incentive alone would not be enough. (Chen et al., 2014) It was interesting that higher workload was associated with better RUM status, though it is not obvious in this study. And we suppose that higher workload might lead to higher pay.

Revenue structure of a health institution represented what the health institution relied on to sustain its operation. For VHCs and THCs, public subsidy might improve RUM while superior outpatient medicine revenue seemed to be in connection with irrational use of medicines. This was consistent in policy logic. Nevertheless, this trend was unable to be witnessed in the CHs. The reasons may be the complex revenue structure of CHs and low proportion of their governmental subsidy and outpatient medicine revenue.

In addition, apart from SREB, the policies related to RUM or NEMS and the relevant trainings appeared to promote RUM.

It is a pity that we were not able to obtain all the organizational indicators we were interested in. There should be other organizational barriers associated with RUM achievement not mentioned in this study. We also believe that the effect of some organizational indicators on RUM in one tier of health institutions could be also generalized to other tiers of health institutions, e.g. zero mark-up policy, EMs outfit and training status.

Chapter 7　Conclusion

To a certain degree, the NEMS in China has taken effect on RUM between 2009 and 2011, but it did not attain to the policy goal and WHO reference standard. Hence it should be developed and further implemented.

At the in-depth stage of the NHCR, the RUM status in the rural areas of western China was unsatisfactory across the regions and the three-tier health network. Excess use of medicines remained popular, and improper polypharmacy and use of antibiotics and injections was the main impediment to RUM achievement, while EMs were not fully used. Besides, medicine expense was very high for people to afford.

A comprehensive evaluation method for overall RUM status was established and could present similar results with SDUIs. Synthetic assessment scores were generated to explore organizational barriers associated with the achievement of RUM as an outcome variable.

Many organizational indicators associated with the achievement of RUM were found. Town-run VHCs had evidently better RUM status. Overstaffed health workers led to irrational use of medicines in VHCs and THCs. Adequate training of RUM and NEMS could improve RUM. SREB, which had been considered a good management policy for public health institutions to eliminate perverse fiscal incentives hence to promote RUM, was a remarkable organizational barrier to achieve RUM. Many other organizational indicators should be also taken into consideration as for potential association with RUM achievement.

7.1　Policy recommendation

The details of implementation of the NEMS and RUM related policies should be drawn, amplified and improved to supervise prescribers' behavior effectively. As an isolated policy will hardly take effect in vast-territory and overpopulated China, dynamically integrated solutions are needed.

It is very essential to keep a watchful eye on sustainable operation of health institutions. As the policies, e.g. zero mark-up policy, tend to restrain medicines abuse, the revenue of health institutions originated from medicines may decrease markedly and they may face financial distress. Therefore, it has set a very high request for governmental fiscal subsidy to improve implementation effect of the policies, especially in the less-developed rural areas of western China. Unfortunately, one of the most widely implemented strategies—SREB failed in THCs and CHs according to our study. This suggests that the government consider its support capacity as well. We believe that, appropriate increasing of medicine price or medicine fee and some financial autonomy of health institutions are not the obstructers to RUM achievement, because on one side, they can help fund health institutions operation and arouse health workers' initiative of providing high-qualified medical services instead of solely pursuing profits if positive balance point is reached, and on other side, they can keep drug-makers providing high-qualified medicines for the market. Moreover, health insurance should be given full play, and its payment, such as capitalization and diagnosis-related groups, should be put into practice to make health resource utilization and medical expenditure control effective and efficient. Besides, non-governmental investments should be exploited. (Charles & Lu, 2011)

In the rural three-tier health service network, the superior health institutions should undertake operational and professional guidance to the inferior ones. Building a more intimate relationship can enhance the service capability of PHIs, and superior health institutions will also benefit from it in terms of reduction of workload, so the quality of health service in rural areas will be improved.

The education of medicine use and medicine policies for both health workers and the public is necessary. On-job training should be offered to health workers at regular and irregular intervals to promote rational prescribing behaviors. And knowledge on medicines should be vigorously disseminated to the public in order to avoid improper use of medicines and boost medication compliance.

A system should be set up to continuously monitor medicine use. The observations of RUM indicators, which can be derived from SDUIs or selected based on actual circumstances in China, should be summarized with some data management approach for medicine use, such as defined daily dose, ABC analysis and VEN analysis. (WHO, 2003b) The most important crux for the system is the absence of a standing official body to gather data throughout the country timely and effectively, and then summarize and report the RUM status to the public. There is a website that engages in this affair, which is named Chinese Monitoring Network for Rational Use of Drugs (www.cnrud.com), and built when the NEMS was launched. However, there has been few updates after 2012. In addition, to make comparable and compatible data for consistent study on the RUM status, we suggest a standard be established for producing, collecting and transferring data. A nationally unified database for electronic data capture is an option.

7.2   Limitations

The results of this study should be interpreted in the light of some limitations. Firstly, the source data was collected through various ways, of which the consistency might compromised; some information about the RUM indicators and organizational characteristics we interested in was not contained in the second hand data, so partial and incomplete analysis was inevitable. However, recognized and scientific methods of data cleaning and imputation were used to cut loss of data quality. Secondly, SDUIs for patient care were studied. Thus we could not conclude the RUM status from patients' perspective. Then, the whole picture of the RUM status and its organizational barriers, and RUM for specific medicine categories, e.g. antibiotics, or for specific therapeutic areas were not fully elucidated. Fourthly, the use of PCA was less effective to calculate a comprehensive evaluation score for comparing with other studies, because the model was established by the normalized data for the study itself. We just throw out a minnow to catch a whale for discussing a viable method to evaluate the overall complexion of RUM and compare the RUM status among the objects within a single study. In spite of these limitations, there are some important findings on the RUM status and its organizational barriers under the context of NHCR, e.g. providing the evidence of SREB failure on achieving RUM. Besides, some of the limitations can be simply patched in future work.

7.3　Perspectives of future work

This study is can be further improved. The study focus can be put on the use of antibiotics and injections, or the use of medicines of some specific therapeutic areas. Health institutions in urban areas as well as in eastern and central regions were out of scope of the study, and the RUM status and its organizational barriers there can be investigated by repeating this research. Tertiary hospitals and inpatient prescriptions can be involved in future study. Should the dynamic data be consistent and applicable, researches on RUM in the recent years can be conducted preferably. Besides, more statistical methods to establish a comprehensive evaluation approach for RUM can be tested as well.

References

Ahmed, S. M. & Islam, Q. S. (2012). Availability and rational use of drugs in primary healthcare facilities following the national drug policy of 1982: is Bangladesh on right track? *J Health Popul Nutr*, 30(1).

Allander, T., Tammi, M. T., Eriksson, M. et al. (2005). Cloning of a human parvovirus by molecular screening of respiratory tract samples. *Proc Natl Acad Sci USA*, 102(36).

Aronson J. K. (2004). Rational prescribing, appropriate prescribing. *British Journal of Clinical Pharmacology*, 57.

Asscher, A. W., Parr, G. D. & Whitmarsh, V. B. (1995). Towards the safer use of medicines. *BMJ*, 311(7011).

Awad, A. I., Ball, D. E. & Eltayeb, I. B. (2007). Improving rational drug use in Africa: the example of Sudan. *East Mediterr Health J*, 13(5).

Bajis, S., Van den Bergh, R., Bruycker, D. et al. (2014). Antibiotic use in a district hospital in Kabul, Afghanistan: are we overprescribing? *Public Health Action*, 4(4).

Bashrahil, K. A. (2010). Indicators of rational drug use and health services in Hadramout, Yemen. *East Mediterr Health J*, 16(2).

Bond, C. A., Cynthia L, R. & Todd, F. (2002). Clinical pharmacy services, hospital pharmacy staffing, and medication errors in United States hospitals. *Pharmacotherapy*, 22(2).

Brudon, P., Rainhorn, J. & Reich, M. R. (1999). *Indicators for monitoring national drug policies. A practical manual* (2nd edn.). Geneva: WHO.

Cao, Y. (2014). The status and effect study of the essential medicine policy. PhD dissertation, Shandong University.

Freeman, C. W. & Boynton, X. L. (2011). *Implementing health care reform policies in China*. Washington D. C: Center for Strategic and International Studies.

Chaudhury, R. R., Parameswar, R., Gupta, U. et al. (2005). Quality medicines for the poor: experience of the Delhi programme on rational use of drugs. *Health Policy & Plan*, 20(2).

Chen, F., Sun, Z. & Zhao, Y. (2006). Problems and counter-measures of concentrated tendering procurement of medicines. *Practical Journal of Medicine & Pharmacy*, 23(2).

Chen, J. G. & Wang, Y. Z. (2010). *China social security system development report*. Beijing: Social Sciences Academic Press.

Chen, L., Wang, S., Wang, Q. et al. (2002). Fieldsurvey of international RDU indicators. *Evaluation and Analysis of Drug-use in Hospital of China*, 2(6).

Chen, L., Wang, S., Wang, Q. et al. (2003a). Field Survey of International RDU Indicators.*China Pharmacy*, 14(3).

Chen, L., Wang, S., Wang, Q. et al. (2003b). Multicenter international indicator control study, field survey for the rational use of drugs—field investigation. *Chinese Journal of Hospital Pharmacy*, 23(7).

Chen, M. S., Wang, L. J., Chen, W. et al. (2014). Does economic incentive matter for rational use of medicine? China's experience from the essential medicines program. *Pharmacoeconomics*, 32(3).

Chen, W., Ye, L., Ying, X. et al. (2007). National essential medicine policy under the context of New Health Care Reform. *Chinese Health*, 13(3).

Chen, Y. (2011). Study on monitoring indicators for rational drug use in community health centers in one district of Shanghai. PhD dissertation, Fudan University.

Chen, Z. (2009). Launch of the health-care reform plan in China. *Lancet*, 373(9672).

Chen, Z., Shi, L. & Guan, X. (2013). Investigation and survey of essential drugs provision and use in primary health care institutions from some areas in China. *China Pharmacy*, 24(3).

Cheng, X. (2003). *Health Economics*. Beijing: People's Medical

Publishing House.

China Public Health and Family Planning Statistical Yearbook. (2015a). Beijing: Pecking Union Medical College Press.

China Public Health and Family Planning Statistical Yearbook. (2015b). Beijing: Pecking Union Medical College Press.

China Public Health and Family Planning Statistical Yearbook. (2015c). Beijing: Peking Union Medical College Press.

China CPG. (2009). Opinions of the CPC Central Committee and the State Council on deepening the health care system reform. <http://www.gov.cn/jrzg/2009-04/06/content_1278721.htm>

China MoH. (1992). Formulating a scheme on national essential medicines policy. Beijing: Drug Administration Department, Ministry of Health of China.

China MoH. (2002). The outline for development of rural primary health care in China, 2001-2010. < http://www. moh. gov. cn/zwgkzt/pzcqgh/200804/31123.shtml>

China MoH. (2009). Briefing of the health development in China. <http://www.moh.gov.cn/zwgkzt/pnb/201001/45652.shtml>

China NHFPC. (2012). Essential Medicines List 2012 released. <http://www. moh. gov. cn/mohywzc/s3582/201303/b058a4edf14e4dc9a1f6f0f0c71a2cce.shtml>

China NHFPC. (2014). Statistical bulletin of the health development in China. < http://www. nhfpc. gov. cn/guihuaxxs/s10742/201511/191ab1d8c5f240e8b2f5c81524e80f19.shtml>

Christensen, R. (1990). A strategy for the improvement of prescribing and drug use in rural facilities on Uganda. Uganda Essential Drug Management Programme.

De Silva, W. A. S. (1981). *Essential drugs.* Sri Lanka.

Dong, L. F., Yan, H. & Wang, D. L. (2011). Drug prescribing indicators in village health clinics across 10 provinces of Western China. *Fam Pract*, 28(1).

Fabrigar, L. R., Wegener, D. T., MacCallum, R., et al. (1999). Evaluating the use of exploratory factor analysis in psychological research. *Psychological Methods*, 4(3).

Fan, C., Zhang, B. & Zhang, L. (2012). Injection safety assessments in two Chinese provinces, 2001-2009: progress and remaining challenges. *International Health*, 4(4).

Feng, S., Li, L., Mu, X. et al. (2012). Problems and Countermeasures of China's Western Human Resources for Health. *Chinese Primary Health Care*, 26(9).

Fu, W., Sun, Y., Sun, J. et al. (2004). Analysis on the rational use of medicines and its control measures in rural township health Centers. *Chinese Health Economics*, 23(6).

Ghimire, S., Nepal, S., Bhandari, S. et al. (2009). A prospective surveillance of drug prescribing and dispensing in a teaching hospital in Western Nepal. *Journal of Pakistan Medical Association*, 59(10).

Grimshaw, J. M. , Thomas, R. E., MacLennan, G. et al. (2004). Effectiveness and efficiency of guideline dissemination and implementation strategies. *Health Technol Assess*, 8(6).

Guan, A., Li, L., Sheng, L. et al. (2007). On-the-spot survey of rational use of drugs in our hospital using selected indicators. *China Pharmacy*, 18(25).

Guan, X. & Shi, L. (2009a). Research on China essential medicine system. *Journal of China Pharmaceutical*, 44(2).

Guan, X. & Shi, L. (2009b). Research on establishment of national essential drug policy in China. *Chinese Pharmaceutical Journal*, 44(2).

Han, Z., Gao, M. & Shen, H. (2008). The relationship between national essential medicine system and basic medical insurance system. *China Pharmaceuticals*, 17(22).

Harvey, K. J., Stewrt, R., Hemming, M. et al. (1986). Educational antibiotic advertising. *The Medical Journal of Australia*, 145(1).

Hitchen, L. (2006). Adverse drug reactions result in 250,000 UK admissions a year. *BMJ*, 332(7550).

Hoen, E . (2002).TRIPS, pharmaceutical patents and access to essential medicines: a long way from Seattle to Doha. *Chicago Journal of International Law*, 1.

Hogerzeil, H. V. (1995). Promoting rational prescribing: an international perspective. *British Journal of Clinical Pharmacology*, 39(1).

Hogerzeil, H. V., Walker, G. J., Sallami, A O. et al. (1989). Impact of an essential drugs programme on availability and rational use of drugs. *Lancet*, 1(8630).

Howard, N. J. & Laing, R. O. (1991). Changes in the world health organization essential drug list. *Lancet*, 338.

Hoyle, M. H. (1973). Transformations: an introduction and a bibliography. *International Statistical Review*, 41(2).

Hu, J., Chang, P. & Yuan, H. (2011). Investigation on the outpatient use of injections in primary hospital. *Clinical Rational Drug Use*, 4(6C).

Huang, Y. (2007). Establishment and development of the national system for basic drugs. *China Pharmaceuticals*, 16(24).

Huang, Y. & Zhou, Y. (2011). Analysis of medicine use for 262 cases of infantile diarrhea. *Journal of North Pharmacy*, 8(12).

Isah, A. O., Ross-Degnan, D., Quick, J. et al. (2006). The development of standard values for the WHO drug use prescribing indicators. Paper presented at the International Conference on Improving Use of Medicines, Geneva.

JE., I. -H. (1993). Essential Drugs. *Ann Med*, 25(1).

Jiang, L., Wang, J. & Jin, D. (2005). Rational medicine use in the whole course of pharmaceutical care. *Herald of Medicine*, 24(6).

Jin, S. H. (2009). Medication prescription for acute upper respiratory infection in community health services in Haikou. *Chinese General Practice*, 12(22).

Johnson, J. A. & Bootman, J. L. (1995). Drug-related morbidity and mortality. A cost-of-illness model. *Arch Intern Med*, 155(18).

Kaiser, H. F. & Rice, J. (1974). Little Jiffy, Mark IV. *Educational and Psychological Measurement*, 34.

Ke, J. (2008). Investigation of medicine use for infantile diarrhea. *Strait Pharmaceutical Journal*, 20(4).

Kenya MMS & Kenya_MPHS. (2009). Access to Essential Medicines in Keny: Health Facility Survey. Nairobi: Ministry of Medical Services and Ministry of Public Health and Sanitation, Republic of Kenya.

Keohavong, B., Syhakhang, L., Sengaloundeth, S. et al. (2006). Rational use of drugs: prescribing and dispensing practices at public health facilities in Lao PDR. *Pharmacoepidemiol Drug Saf*, 15(5).

Khan, M. I. & Ara, N. (2011). Promoting Rational Prescribing Among Medical Practitioners. *Bangladesh Medical Journal*, 40(2).

Kleinke, J. D. (2001). The price of progress: prescription drugs in the health care market. *Health Affairs*, 20(5).

Kuang, Z., Chen, J., Kuang, Y. et al. (2013). Survey and analysis of international indicators of rational drug use in outpatients of a hospital in 2012. *China Pharmacy*, 24(42).

Laing, R., Waning, B., Gray, A. et al. (2003). 25 years of the WHO essential medicines lists: progress and challenges. *The Lancet*, 361(9370).

Lazarou, J., Pomeranz, B. H. & Corey, P. N. (1998). Incidence of adverse drug reactions in hospitalized patients: a meta-analysis of prospective studies. *JAMA*, 279(15).

Levy, S. B. (2005). Antibiotic resistance—the problem intensifies. *Adv Drug Deliv Rev*, 57(10).

Li, C., Li, S. & Yang, Y. (2011). Study on the WHO evaluation method of rational use of drugs in medical institutions. *China Licensed Pharmacist*, 9(12).

Li, D., Wang, Y., Wang, J. et al. (2015). Analysis of current administration of essential drugs and study on corresponding coping measures for medical institutions in Xinjiang area. *Chinese Journal of Hospital Pharmacy*, 4(35).

Li, J.,Zhang, X. & Wang, H. (2013). The meaningful use of EMR in Chinese hospitals: a case study on curbing antibiotic abuse. *Journal of Medical Systems*, 37(2).

Li, T., Liang, W., Yu, L. et al. (2012). The comparative study on rational use of drugs in primary health institutions before and after the implementation of essential medicine system. *China Pharmaceuticals*, 21(14).

Li, Y. (2011). The status and effect study of the policy implementation of essential drug in Chinese city community health institutions. PhD dissertation, Huazhong University of Science & Technology.

Li, Y., Xu, J., Wang, F. et al. (2012). Overprescribing in China, driven by financial incentives, results in very high use of antibiotics, injections, and corticosteroids. *Health Aff (Millwood)*, 31(5).

Lindtjørn, B. (1987). Essential drug list in a rural hospital. Does it have any influence on drug prescription? *Tropical Doctor*, 17(4).

Liu, J.,Qian, L. & Zhang, X. (2003). "Delhi Model" and essential medicine promotion. *Foreign Medical Sciences. Social Medicine Section*, 6(2).

Liu, Y. & Gao, J. (2006). Hormone abuse investigation: use of hormones without indications, excessive use of hormones, reducing dosage or stopping use of hormones unexpectedly are very common. *Capital Medicine*, 12.

Liu, Y. & Gao, J. (2007). Investigation on hormones abuse. China pharmaceuticals. *China Pharmaceuticals*, 16(4).

Lofgren, H. & Boer, R. D. (2004). Pharmaceuticals in Australia: developments in regulation and governance. *Soc Sci Med*, 58(12).

Lv, Z., Guo, X., Zhong, H. et al. (2009). Analysis of medicine use for emergency treatment of upper respiratory infection. *Chinese Journal of Nosocomiology*, 19(18).

Mamdani, M. (1992). *Early initiatives in essential drugs policy.* London: Zed Books.

Manasee, H. R. (1989). Medication use in an imperfect world: drug misadventuring as an issue of public policy, Part 1. *Am J Hosp Pharm*, 46(5).

Mao, W., Zhang, L., Chen, W. et al. (2013). Allocation and utilization of essential Medicines at primary health care institutions. *Chinese Health Resources*, 16(2).

Mardan, A., Gulibahar, K., Ayiguli et al. (2014). Analysis on Utilization of Health Services in Township Health Centers in Impoverished Counties in Xinjiang. *Chinese Journal of Primary Medicine and Pharmacy*, 21(23).

Meng, R. (2009). *The Discipline of Pharmacy Administration* (2nd edn.). Beijing: China Science Publishing & Media Ltd.

MSH. (2012). Promoting rational prescribing. Boston: Management Sciences for Health.

Pirmohamed, M., James, S., Meakin, S. et al. (2004). Adverse drug reactions as cause of admission to hospital: prospective analysis of 18,820 patients. *BMJ*, 329.

Nie, C., Yao, L., Cui, B. et al. (2002). Analysis on the irrational use of drugs in pilot areas. *Chinese Primary Health Care*, 16(4).

Nie, C., Yao, L., Lu, Z. et al. (2002). Review of MoH & UNICEF program on norming rural primary health workers' prescribing behaviors. *Chinese Primary Health Care*, 16(3).

Norman, R. (2001). National drug policy: implications of the tough on drugs' ideology. *Collegian*, 8(4).

Odusanya. (2004). Drug use indicators at a secondary health care facility in Lagos, Nigeria. *Journal of Community Medicine & Primary Health Care*, 16.

Ogendi, P. O. (2011). Access to essential medicines and the utilisation of compulsory licensing and parallel importation in Kenya and South Africa. Master's dissertation, University Of Nairobi.

Pavin, M., Nurgozhin, T., Hafner, G. et al. (2003). Prescribing practices of rural primary health care physicians in Uzbekistan. *Trop Med Int Health*, 8(2).

Pereira Gomes, V., Melo da Silva, K., Oliveira Chagas., S. et al. (2015). Off-label and unlicensed utilization of drugs in a Brazilian pediatric hospital. *Farm Hosp*, 39(3).

Polit, D. & Beck, C. (2012). *Nursing research: generating and assessing evidence for nursing practice* (9th edn.). Philadelphia: Wolters Klower Health, Lippincott Williams & Wilkins.

Qu, J. (2004). Rational drug use in hospital pharmacy. *Pharmaceutical Care and Research*, 4(1).

Quick, J., Rankin, J., Laing, R. et al. (1997). *Managing drug supply* (2nd edn.). West Hartford: Kumarian Press.

Reynolds, L. & McKee, M. (2009). Factors influencing antibiotic prescribing in China: an exploratory analysis. *Health Policy*, 90(1).

Rishi, R. K., Sangeeta, S., Surendra, K. et al. (2003). Prescription audit: experience in Garhwal (Uttaranchal), India. *Tropical Doctor*, 33(2).

Shaw, P. (2003). *Multivariate statistics for the environmental sciences*. London: Hodder-Arnold.

Shen, L. (2003). Brief introduction to Australia's national drug policy. *Shanghai Medical & Pharmaceutical Journal*, 24(6).

Simonsen, L., Kane, A., Lloyd, J. et al. (1999). Unsafe injections in the developing world and transmission of bloodborne pathogens: a review. *Bull World Health Organ*, 77(10).

Song, Y. (2013). Effect of national essential medicine system in China—emprical study on rural primary health centers from four provinces. PhD dissertation, University of Macau.

Su, Y., Su, C. & Yang, J. (2008). Analysis on antibiotic use rationality in a hospital in the first half year of 2006. *Chinese Journal of Hospital Pharmacy*, 28(16).

Suleman, F. (1997). The concept of rational drug use. *South African Medical Journal*, 87(4).

Sun, S. (2010, Oct. 12). Abuse of antibiotics causes more harm than bacteria. *Yang Cheng Evening News*.

Tang, J. (1998). *The international network for rational use of drugs newsletters: Chinese yearbook*. Beijing: Science and Technology of China Press.

Tang, J., Chen, X., Tan, J. et al. (1995). The international investigation indicators for rational drug use. *China Pharmacy*, 6(4).

Tang, J. & Li, J. (2011). Successful health care reform requiring strong support of rational drug use regulation. *China Pharmacy*, 22(37).

Tang, J. & Yuan, J. (2010). Practicality and interdependence of essential drug system, primary health care and rational drug use system. *China Pharmacy*, 21(12).

Tang, Y., Zhang, X., Yang, C. et al. (2013). Application of propensity scores to estimate the association between government subsidy and injection use in primary health care institutions in China. *BMC Health Serv Res*, 13.

Tett, S. E. (2004). A perspective on Australia's national medicine policy. *Can J Clin Pharmacol*, 11(1).

Tian, L. & Yu, P. (2005). Discussion on the irrational drug use and the countermeasures in China. *China Pharmacy*, 16(16).

Troup, R. G. (1989). What influences doctors' prescribing? *Journal of the Royal College of General Practitioners*, 39(323).

Tu, X. (2013). Medicine utilization of outpatient in a tertiary level hospital in Wuhan city. PhD dissertation, Huazhong University of Science and Technology.

Vaananen, M. H., Pietila, K. & Airaksinen, M. (2006). Self-medication with antibiotics—does it really happen in Europe? *Health Policy*, 77(2).

van Roosmalen, M. S., Braspenning, J. C. C., De Smet, P. A. G. M. et al. (2007). Antibiotic prescribing in primary care: first choice and restrictive prescribing are two different traits. *Qual Saf Health Care*, 16(2).

Verhoef, J., Fluit, A. C., Jansen, W. T. M. et al. (2005). Resistance: A sensitive issue. Strategic council on resistance in Europe. *International Journal of Risk and Safety in Medicine*, 17(3/4).

Wan, C., Yang, Z., Wei, L. et al. (2014). Effect analysis on implementation of the national system for basic drugs in township central hospitals of Jiujiang City. *China Modern Medicine*, 21(29).

Wang, J. (2009). Investigation and analysis of drugs irrationally used in outpatient prescriptions. *China Pharmaceuticals*, 18(22).

Wang, J., Gu, J. & Wang, X. (2006). The rational medicine use of infantile Diarrhea. *Chinese Community Doctors*, 22(10).

Wang, K., Lin, Y. & Dong, H. (2000). Causes of the unduly rapid growth of drug expenses in China and countermeasures. *Chin J Hosp Admin*, 16(5).

Wang, Q., Wang, Y., Li, S. et al. (2002). Multi-centerintervention research on selected drug use indicators. *Chinese Pharmaceutical Journal*, 37(3).

Wang, Q., Wang, Y. & Ma, J. (2004). A glance at the second international conference on improving use of medicines. *China Pharmacy*, 15(6).

Wang, Y., Wang, H., Wang, S., Shi, L. et al. (2002). Multi-center controlled study on rational use of medicine with prescription analysis by international indicators, *Chinese Journal of Pharmaco Epiolemiology*, 11(2).

Wei, J., Zou, M. & Li, Z. (2014). Current situation of the rational use of drugs in outpatients in Shenzhen Traditional Chinese Medicine Hospital and related influential factors. *Pharmaceutical Care and Research*, 14(5).

Wei, Y. & Zeng, R. (2016). Study on outpatient rational drug use and related factors in a hospital in Shenzhen. *Journal of North Pharmacy*, 13(1).

White T. J., Arakelian A. & Rho, J. P. (1999). Counting the costs of drug-related adverse events. *Pharmacoeconomics*, 15(5).

WHO. (1985). Report of the conference of experts on the rational use of drugs. Nairobi.

WHO. (1987). The rational use of drugs.

WHO. (1988). Guidelines for developing national drug policies.

WHO. (1993). How to investigate drug use in health facilities: selected drug use indicators.

WHO. (2000a). Problems of irrational use of drugs.

WHO. (2000b). The use of essential drugs: report of a WHO expert committee. Technical report series no 895.

WHO. (2002a). Essential drugs monitor.

WHO. (2002b). Essential medicines list and WHO model formulary.

WHO. (2002c). Procedure to update and disseminate the WHO model list of essential medicines document EB109/8 (Annex).

WHO. (2002d). Promoting rational use of medicines: core components.

WHO. (2002e). Safety of medicines—A guide to detecting and reporting adverse drug reactions—Why health professionals need to take actions.

WHO. (2003a). Adherence to long-term therapies: evidence for action.

WHO. (2003b). Drug and the rapeutics committees—A practical guide.

WHO. (2004). The world medicine situation 2004.

WHO. (2006). Using indicators to measure country pharmaceutical situations: fact book on WHO level I and level II monitoring indicators.

WHO. (2007a). Resolutions of the sixtieth World Health Assembly.

WHO. (2007b). WHO operational package for monitoring and assessing country pharmaceutical situations: guide for coordinators and data collectors.

WHO. (2009a). Clinical management of human infection with new influenza A(H1N1) virus: initial guidance.

WHO. (2009b). Medicine use in primary care in developing and transitional countries: fact book summarizing results from studies reported between 1990 and 2006.

WHO. (2010a). 10 facts on essential medicines.

WHO. (2010b). Policy, access and rational use (PAR): main challenges and strategic direction.

WHO. (2011a). Antibiotics may lose their power to cure disease.

WHO. (2011b). The world medicine situation.

WHO. Managing drug supply (2nd edn.).

WHO/DAP. (1998). Action programme on essential drugs. Progress of

WHO member states in developing national drug policies and in revising essential drugs lists.

WHO/EDM. (2001). Updating and disseminating the WHO model list of essential drugs: the way forward.

WHO/UNICEF. (1978). Health for all. Paper presented at the International Conference on Primary Health Care, Alma-Alta, USSR.

Willems, D. L. (2001). Balancing rationalities: gatekeeping in health care. *Journal of Medical Ethics*, 27.

Wu, Y. & Jiao, Y. (2010). *Guide to clinical formulation and use of intravenous medicine*. Beijing: People's Medical Publishing House.

Xiao, Y., Wang, J., Shen, P. et al. (2016). Retrospective survey of the efficacy of mandatory implementation of the essential medicine policy in the primary healthcare setting in China: failure to promote the rational use of antibiotics in clinics. *Int J Antimicrob Agents*, 48(4).

Yan, Y., Wang, H., Zhang, X. et al. (2005). Area investigation of rational use of drugs with selected drug use indicators in grade-two hospitals in Shanghai suburbs. *Pharmaceutical Care and Research*, 5(2).

Yang, C., Yang, S., Xiang, X. et al. (2013). Influence of essential medicine system on rational drug use in primary health care institutions in Hubei. *Medicine and Society*, 26(1).

Yang, J. (2006). *Study on evaluation of interventions and strategies to improve use of drugs in rural areas of China*. Master's dissertation, Huazhong University of Science and Technology.

Yang, L., Liu, C., Ferrier, J. A. et al. (2015). Organizational barriers associated with the implementation of national essential medicine policy: across-sectional study of township hospitals in China. *Soc Sci Med*, 145.

Yang, X. (2006). Study on rational use of drugs in 3-level medical organizations in rural areas of western China. PhD dissertation, Huazhong University of Science & Technology.

Yao, L., Jin, J., Cui, B. et al. (2002). Research on norming rural primary health workers' prescribing behaviors in China—Analysis on the irrational use of drugs in the pilot areas. *Chinese Health Economics*, 21(6).

Yoongthong, W., Hu, S., Whitty, J. A. et al. (2012). National drug policies to local formulary decisions in Thailand, China, and Australia: drug listing changes and opportunities. *Value Health*, 15(1).

Yu, D., Ma, Y., Zhang, S. et al. (2011). Problems and countermeasures in implementing national basic medicine system. *Chinese Health Economics*, 30(12).

Yu, G. (2007). Implementation of national essential medicine system, achieving the goal of "everybody enjoys the primary health care". *Shanghai Medical & Pharmaceutical Journal*, 28(3).

Zhang, K.,Ren, Y. & Peng, S. (2001). Rational use of drugs in Xizang Plateau. *The Journal of Pharmaceutical Practice*, 19(2).

Zhang, X. & Zheng, M. (2005). The indicators value of evaluation of rational use of medicines in rural areas. *Chinese Primary Health Care*, 19(12).

Zhang, Y., Li, Z. & Chen, J. (2011). Discussion on the management and development of township health centers. *Acta Universitatis Medicinalis Nanjing (Social Science)*, 12(2).

Zhang, Y. & Zhi, M. (1995). Index system, appraising method for comprehensive appraisal. *J North Jiaotong Univ*, 19.

Zhao, F. & Miao, Y. (2001). Hazard of irrational use of medicines and strategies to ensure rational use of medicines. *Chinese Journal of Misdiagnostics*, 1(1).

Zheng, S., Song, Y., Yin, S. et al. (2014). Impact analysis of national essential medicine system on rational drug use in primary health care institution of Ningxia Hui Autonomous Region. *Chinese Primary Health Care*, 28(8).

Zhou, S. & Yang, X. (2009). Current situation and counter-measures of irrational clinical use of medicines. *Guide of China Medicine*, 7(22).

Zhu, S., Li, Y., Wang, Y. et al. (2009). Analysis of 247 severe adverse drug reaction/event cases. *Chinese Journal of Pharmacovigilance*, 6(10).

Zou, J. (2015). Analysis on the implementation of separation between revenues and expenditures in town hospitals. *Journal of Today Health*, 14(8).